When Symptoms Meet
SCIENCE

Team Up with Your Doctor
Without Knowing Latin or Greek
(*A Patient's Guidebook for Effective Medical Consultation*)

When Symptoms Meet
SCIENCE

Tiny Nair
MD DM FACC FRCP
Head
Department of Cardiology
PRS Hospital
Thiruvananthapuram, Kerala, India

Foreword

HK Chopra

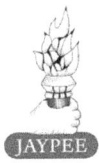

JAYPEE BROTHERS MEDICAL PUBLISHERS
The Health Sciences Publisher
New Delhi | London

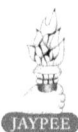 **Jaypee Brothers Medical Publishers (P) Ltd**

Headquarters
EMCA House
23/23-B, Ansari Road, Daryaganj
New Delhi 110 002, India
Landline: +91-11-23272143
+91-11-23272703, +91-11-23282021
+91-11-23245672
E-mail: jaypee@jaypeebrothers.com

Corporate Office
Jaypee Brothers Medical Publishers (P) Ltd.
4838/24, Ansari Road, Daryaganj
New Delhi 110 002, India
Phone: +91-11-43574357
Fax: +91-11-43574314
E-mail: jaypee@jaypeebrothers.com

Corporate Office
Jaypee Brothers Medical Publishers (P) Ltd.
4838/24, Ansari Road, Daryaganj
New Delhi 110 002, India
Phone: +91-11-43574357
E-mail: jaypee@jaypeebrothers.com

EU GPSR Authorised Representative
Logos Europe, 9 rue Nicolas Poussin
17000, La Rochelle, France
Phone: +33 (0) 6 67 93 73 78
E-mail: Contact@logoseurope.eu

Website: www.jaypeebrothers.com
Website: www.jaypeedigital.com

© 2024, Jaypee Brothers Medical Publishers

The views and opinions expressed in this book are solely those of the original contributor(s)/author(s) and do not necessarily represent those of editor(s) or publisher of the book.

All rights reserved. No part of this publication may be reproduced, stored or transmitted in any form or by any means, electronic, mechanical, photocopying, recording or otherwise, without the prior permission in writing of the publishers.

All brand names and product names used in this book are trade names, service marks, trademarks or registered trademarks of their respective owners. The publisher is not associated with any product or vendor mentioned in this book.

Medical knowledge and practice change constantly. This book is designed to provide accurate, authoritative information about the subject matter in question. However, readers are advised to check the most current information available on procedures included and check information from the manufacturer of each product to be administered, to verify the recommended dose, formula, method and duration of administration, adverse effects and contraindications. It is the responsibility of the practitioner to take all appropriate safety precautions. Neither the publisher nor the author(s)/editor(s) assume any liability for any injury and/or damage to persons or property arising from or related to use of material in this book.

This book is sold on the understanding that the publisher is not engaged in providing professional medical services. If such advice or services are required, the services of a competent medical professional should be sought.

Every effort has been made where necessary to contact holders of copyright to obtain permission to reproduce copyright material. If any have been inadvertently overlooked, the publisher will be pleased to make the necessary arrangements at the first opportunity.

Inquiries for bulk sales may be solicited at: jaypee@jaypeebrothers.com

When Symptoms Meet Science / Tiny Nair

First Edition: **2024**

ISBN: 978-93-5696-689-5

Dedication

This book is dedicated to
my wife *Deepa*,
my daughter *Parvathy,* and
my son *Akash*.

Why This Book?

The spectrum of a doctor–patient relationship ranges from one filled with utmost humility and gratitude to one frothing with frustration, anger, and vengeance. It is sometimes rock-solid, undisturbed by a 10 richter-scale earthquake of a deadly disease, while at times as fragile as a piece of glass, shattering at the slightest impact, ending up in breach of trust, a lawsuit.

Or worse, physical violence.

Instead of sitting *across* the table, is it possible that the doctor and the patient sit on the *same side* as a team, facing their common enemy, the disease?

Yes, it is indeed a disruptive concept. We are *not* talking about doctor–patient cordiality but one step beyond. We are talking about a scenario where we team up together for a win-win situation.

This book looks at a very narrow window of doctors' consultation, something that has traditionally been neglected, and how to improve it for the benefit of both.

After all, the common enemy is disease and ill-health.

Let the patient's *symptom* meet and team up with the *science* of medicine.

Wisdom for the Doctor

"The biggest challenge of medicine is to watch terminally ill patient die, knowing that you have nothing else to do, while telling him not to worry".

Wisdom for Everyone
including the Doctor

You might be extremely pious, hardworking, talented, and gifted person.

You might be exceptional, near genius.

Still, you might get up tomorrow morning with a diagnosis of cancer, stroke, or heart attack. It is not rare.

55,000 *nice* people got a new diagnosis of cancer; 40,000 *talented* people woke up with a weakness of one side resulting from stroke; and 35,000 *hardworking* people got out of bed with an unexplained chest heaviness turning out to be a heart attack, in one single day. For no fault of theirs.

All that number in one single day, globally.

None of them went to bed thinking that they would be the victim.

For them, the unwatched "YouTube" or the ready-to-upload "Tik-tok" video or the "Insta post" became irrelevant.

"Ohh God, if only my disease went away, I would be so lucky and happy", they all lament.

Let us presume today you do not have any of these dreaded maladies.

Then why aren't you happy?

Do you want to *get* such a disease, *get cured*, to be happy?

Is your doctor serious or funny?

Strict or casual?

Starched white coat or soft-faded denim?

Does he let out a staccato of opinion from the atria of his larynx or releases measured amount of wisdom from the ventricle of his heart?

Why should you bother about it?

And why the hell should you try to make him happy.

Or, make him smile?

And why should you team up with him?

Symptoms meet science.

Foreword

It is a great pleasure and honor indeed for me in writing the Foreword for the need-based state-of-art book with brainstorming, mindboggling, and scintillating thought-provoking contents in *"When Symptoms Meet Science"*, a patient's guidebook for effective medical consultation, authored by my great friend, extraordinary clinical cardiologist Dr Tiny Nair, Head, Department of Cardiology, PRS Hospital, Thiruvananthapuram, Kerala, India. The main theme of this book is to enhance the robust relationship between doctor and patient to beat the disease effectively together. The book highlights on the wisdom of the doctor and everyone around him, including God's grace.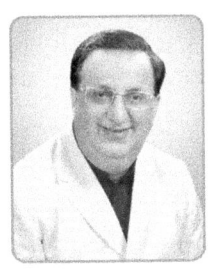

The book's navigation is divided into three parts: Section 1, focusing on doctor's mental algorithm and patient's anxiousness; Section 2, dealing with common pitfalls during the meetings and hilarious stories that end with clear directions; Section 3, the way forward. The "to-do"—right from tomorrow. Section 1 contains 10 chapters including The Science, Setting the Stage, Inside the Doctor's Mind, Specialization and Loss of Family Physician, Accidents and Family Reunion: India is Different, More Insight: East versus West, Kerbside Consult: Right or Wrong? Investigations, and More, Opinion, Option, or Direction, Doctor Relative. Section 2 contains 20 chapters including Timing is Everything, Gas, Doc Scare, Teaching the Doctor, Be Kind, Stab the Lab, Memory Test, Old Records, Bystanders, Gossip, Tests and More Tests, Diagnosis: Yours or Mine? Criticizing the Previous Doctor, Minor Irritants, Loss of Focus, Emotional Blackmail, Warranty, Medical Jargon and Acronym, Medicine Dosage, Walking-in, Allergy, and Fake News. Section 3 contains four chapters including Dress, How to Select a Specialist, Second Opinion, and Tools to Carry.

The chapters are well outlined, organized, and well written with authenticity. The writing style of every chapter is vivid, concise, practical, eloquent, and guideline directed. The clinical examples are exhilarating and thought provoking with meaningful messages.

Dr Tiny Nair is an epitome of devotion, dedication, dynamism, philosophy, and humanity all in one. He is also an apostle of elegance and generosity in every aspect of expressions in this book. He is also an embodiment of compassion, selfless service, sacrifice, healing, humility, humanity, and hope and a crusader of victory and vision. His book nurtures positivity during crisis and emergency care.

Foreword

I congratulate Dr Tiny Nair for accomplishing this extraordinary brilliant achievement of amalgamation of great clinical relevance in the realm of *"When Symptoms Meet Science"* with integration of physical orchestra, emotional orchestra, neurohormonal and biochemical orchestra, genetic and epigenetic orchestra, and quantum orchestra in human beings.

May I appeal to each and everyone to read, understand, and practice all, mentioned by Dr Tiny Nair in this unique book for enhancing our wisdom connecting doctor–patient relationship.

I wish this book *"When Symptoms Meet Science"* a great success to impact locally, focally, and globally.

> *"The good physician treats the disease; the great physician treats the patient who has the disease and a super great physician prevents the disease by enhancing the Doctor–Patient relationship".*

HK Chopra
Chief Cardiologist, Medanta Moolchand Heart Institute
Chairman CME, Moolchand Medcity, New Delhi
President, World Wellness Foundation, WHA
Country Head, American Heart Association
Chairman, KDC Instant Healthcare India LLP
Editor-in-Chief, Top 14 Focused Textbooks of Cardiology
Editor-in-Chief, 40 Handbooks in Cardiology and Medicine
National Awardee, DST, Government of India
A national Stamp released GOI, for focused Textbook of Cardiology
National Past President, Cardiology Society of India (CSI) and
Indian Academy of Echocardiography (IAE)
Former Editor in Chief, IHJ & JIAE
Published 1,485 Articles in Various National and
International Journals and Textbooks
Worked at Ceders Sinai, Medical Centre, UCLA, USA
University of Alabama, UAB, USA

Preface

Dunning–Kruger syndrome

On a cold January afternoon, 1995, McArthur Wheeler and Clifton Johnson walked into the cash counter of the Mellon Bank at Swissvale, Pittsburgh, pointed a semiautomatic gun at the cashier, and walked away with 5,200 USD cash. Before leaving, Wheeler looked straight at the CCTV camera and smiled. He was sure that his face will not be recognized by the camera because he had dabbed a special formula on his face, *lemon juice*. Both the robbers' smiling pictures were beamed over TV screens within hours of the crime. They were promptly tracked down and arrested.

"But I wore *lemon juice* on my face", was the surprised response of the robber as he was being handcuffed.

It seems his friend had told him that dabbing *lemon juice* on the face makes you unrecognizable on a CCTV camera. He tried smearing some on his face and photographed himself on a polaroid camera and got a blank print, confirming his belief. Obviously, his camera film was defective.

While the whole world laughed at their comical act, and labeled them as dumb, Professor David Dunning and his student Justin Kruger at the Cornell University thought otherwise. The reason why they overestimated their ability to rob a bank was their low skill level. *Dunning–Kruger effect* is defined as overestimation of skill by a person with low skill set, and it holds good for every profession.

I had just graduated from medical school and finished internship and while rest of my friends were dusting their old notes and contemplating study, I made it through the postgraduate (PG) entrance. With a white coat, a black stethoscope, and an inflated ego, I joined the Government Medical College, Trivandrum, as one of the youngest PG students in medicine. I believed that I was good. I was not boastful but felt confidant and certainly proud of my achievement.

The patient in the ward suddenly became breathless. Oxygen and IV line were started, and I jumped into action. But the man was sinking, becoming more and more breathless. We put him in a trolley and fast forward to the intensive coronary care unit (ICCU). I was sure that he was suffering from a heart failure and needed to be connected to a ventilator.

In the mele, one stern female voice said, "Doctor, could you hold on for a moment?" The elderly nurse-in-charge of the ICCU, watching all the drama, came forward with a long forceps in hand. With one swift move, she opened the patient's mouth and pulled out a wired denture form the patient's mouth. Immediately, the patient became quiet and started breathing normally. It was a simple case of aspirated artificial denture that chocked his windpipe. Treated by a set of pseudoconfident, low-skilled doctors, who overestimated their skill, he was saved at the nick of time by an experienced nurse.

Today, years later, I still remember the incident but in a different perspective. This was another young man, a computer professional, who had seen me with high blood pressure, diabetes, and high cholesterol; he had a bad family history, with multiple close relatives suffering heart attacks. I had talked to him and explained as to how important it was to take care of those risk factors as I wrote his prescription. The next time I saw him was 3 years later, at the emergency room (ER) with severe chest pain. ECG showed a massive heart attack, which he mistook as gas.

He had never taken medicines that I had prescribed. He had a skyscraper-high blood sugar, a cloud-hugging cholesterol level, and stratospheric blood pressure number.

"Why did you not take medicines?", I asked.

"Doctor, I always google search and read everything before taking decisions. I read and found out that blood pressure and cholesterol medicines can create kidney and liver problem and memory loss. So, I avoided them. I take green tea, food supplements, and antioxidants. They are very safe, you see".

I did see the connection.

Dunning and Kruger were wrong. It is not just that people with poor skill level who overestimate their skill. People sporting white coat with black stethoscope speaking *Greek* and *Latin*, as well as those conversing in *Java*, tweaking a *Python*, and sleep-off hugging a laptop, are also vying to enter the elite club.

Tiny Nair

Confusion

"Flick-knife-attack" does not necessarily happen in the dark alley outside a nightclub, neither do "hippo-defense" show up in the swamps of Africa. These are exotic names of "moves", in the game of chess, created by grandmasters. In the same line, "trigger-finger" or "tennis-elbow" is not restricted to a gun-totting cowboy or a Wimbledon contestant, but ailments found loitering outside the doctors' clinic. Look carefully, and you would find an uncanny similarity between the "high-IQ" grandmaster and the average "family" doctor.

The grandmaster sits quiet in front of a chessboard, seemingly doing nothing, intermittently moving a small piece now and then. But be it a novice or a grandmaster, there are only 20 possible "first" moves in chess.

To a parent there are just two reasons as to why a kid catches a fever: Either playing in the rain or eating ice-cream. They come to see the doctor with a confirmed diagnosis in mind, for a legal prescription of paracetamol and "doctor-uncles-injection-threat" for repeat offenders. Mostly, the doctor too follows the parental advise. That is the correct "first" move.

"The doctor did nothing and wrote an illegible prescription of paracetamol".

Despite such a humble start with merely 20 first-move options, as the game of chess reaches the fifth move, an enormous 400-billion options spring up, and that is when the game gets more intense.

If the kid's fever does not go away by a week's time, the doctor contemplates the next move; he orders lab tests and scans. If the problem settles in the next few days, the need and motive for all those *unnecessary* tests are doubted; if not, the very first move is questioned.

The assumption that the doctor knows everything at the first glance, and a *simple* antibiotic prescription could have been enough, is as wrong as inferring that the grandmaster knew of the results from the very first move.

Most fevers turn out to be nothing but a nuisance; loss of sleep for the parents, holiday from school, and tasteless *kanji* for a few days for the kid, and everything is forgotten. But serious infections like meningitis, pneumonia, dengue, and leptospirosis start with a *simple* fever. Then there are those more dreaded noninfective causes of fever like hematologic and lymphoreticular malignancies (blood cancers, lymph node cancers) that haunt the physician in the back of his mind, as he balances the options carefully. The next level of tests, like bone marrow aspiration and lymph node biopsy, are invasive, painful, and not complication-free. A parent would have never heard of a lymphoma, a leukemia, or a sarcoidosis and believes that it can never happen to their kids, but the doctors know that they are not uncommon.

Everyone agrees that chess is a high-IQ game but does not understand as to how energy intensive it is. In 1984, grandmaster Anatoly Carpov lost 10 kg weight after a world championship; in 2004, grandmaster Rustam Kasimdzhanov's body weight was reduced by 8.5 kg after just six games. Robert Sapolsky, a neuroscientist from Stanford in an experiment in 2018 on grandmaster Mikhail Antipov, calculated that the grandmaster spent 560 kilocalories during a 2-hour chess competition, matching that of the tennis star Roger Federer playing a 1 hour of tennis singles. Energy-intensive work need not always come dressed in tracksuits and headband. The housewife sitting at home, the schoolteacher taking class online, and the doctor scribbling illegible handwritten prescription are queuing close behind the chess grandmaster, doing invisible calorie-burning.

Sometimes, in the middle of an interesting chess match, the grandmasters suddenly get up, shake hands, and declare it a draw, leaving most of us bewildered. While amateur players can see most available options in front of them, and little beyond, grandmasters in contrast can see much ahead. In an interview, chess prodigy Magnus Carlsen revealed that he could see up to 15 steps ahead with all the possible combinations, but that is after the game has shaped up. The grandmaster can sense an imminent danger much before the king is threatened, and a call of *check* is given.

The doctor too gets the hint of the outcome of a disease much before others, by way of a disturbing biopsy report, an abnormal shadow in a scan, or a deranged blood test. His suggestion on the next course of action often looks out of context, leaving the patient and bystanders bewildered. It is said that, "The biggest challenge of medicine is to watch the terminally ill patient, knowing that you have very little to do, while telling him not to worry".

A human body with 30 trillion cells turns out to be more unpredictable than those 64 black and white "cells" in a chess board. So, unlike chess, the doctor needs *your* help in this game of health.

Check, *mate.*

The overestimation of skills and the complexity of diagnosis lead us to those crucial 5-minute consultation time.

Five Vital Minutes

300,000 milliseconds is a pretty long time. Traveling at the speed of light, you can cover 90 million kilometers in that time span. But once your token number is called and you enter the doctor's clinic, you realize that those 300,000 milliseconds is actually 5 minutes, and that is the average time *a specialist doctor in India spends interacting with you*. GPs are a different level altogether. They are F1, superfast, and clock under 2 minutes. During those crucial 5 minutes, you may get a life-changing news. A failing memory or a fluttering heart, a fast-growing tumor, or a slowly shrinking kidney, this verdict might turn your life upside down.

A correct clinical diagnosis, the right confirmatory tests, and the appropriate treatment are the backbone of "evidence-based" modern medicine, but *missed* diagnosis, *unnecessary* investigations, or *wrong* treatments are not uncommon, though, course correction occurs later.

Traditionally, the doctor is the one who dispenses the verdict, while the client, the patients, accepts it with humility. With educational and legal empowerment and universal availability of powerful internet search engines, the roles are changing fast. Empowered patients come armed with *presumed* diagnosis, check *appropriateness* of investigations, and are sensitized to the side effect of treatment. This led to a different level of patient rights, leading to complaints in news and social media as well as tendency to seek legal help and redressal. But that does not help anyone. Finding fault with the doctor does not cure the disease. A wrong diagnosis, a wasted treatment, an unintended surgical scar, or an inappropriate intervention cannot be *undone* by punishing the guilty or offering financial compensation.

Let us explore a different scenario, one in which the patient can do something more than just receive the prescription or complain about the system. Can he help the doctor in making a right diagnosis or dispense a correct medication or, even better, *join hands* with the medical team for a better journey forward, in every step of decision-making. After all, both the patient and the doctor are trying for the same goal, right diagnosis, and appropriate treatment and cure. Here we are *not* talking about the usual shared decision-making where the doctor shares all the available data or options available, but much beyond that.

Here, the traditionally *passive* "patient" become a pro-active member of the team. Is there an exercise to shed those ugly mental calories of "doctor bashing" if things go wrong and rather be a part of the team themselves? A patient and a doctor joining hands would be the most powerful teamwork we can ever build.

The "time-constrained" doctor with his technical know-how, bogged down by multiple patients, meets the patient focussed to his own problem, sit together, not across the table, but on the same side of the table. They face the disease, the real challenge, as a team.

This is a win-win situation for everyone.

Navigation

This book is divided in three sections.

Section 1: Two Way Traffic
It deals with the background of clinical interaction. This is meant to clarify both the patients' and the doctors' perspective. It deals with how the doctors' mental algorithm works and also how the anxious patient feels.

Section 2: Real Life
It deals with common pitfalls during the meetings. Hilarious stories end with a clear direction.

Section 3: To-do List
The way forward. The "to-do"—right from tomorrow.

Contents

SECTION 1: TWO WAY TRAFFIC

CHAPTER 1:	The Science	3
CHAPTER 2:	Setting the Stage	5
CHAPTER 3:	Inside the Doctor's Mind	10
CHAPTER 4:	Specialization and Loss of Family Physician	12
CHAPTER 5:	Accidents and Family Reunion: India is Different	14
CHAPTER 6:	More Insight: East versus West	17
CHAPTER 7:	Kerb-side Consult: Right or Wrong?	20
CHAPTER 8:	Investigations, and More	23
CHAPTER 9:	Opinion, Option, or Direction	24
CHAPTER 10:	Doctor Relative	26

SECTION 2: REAL LIFE

CHAPTER 11:	Timing is Everything	29
CHAPTER 12:	Gas	31
CHAPTER 13:	Doc Scare	33
CHAPTER 14:	Teaching the Doctor	34
CHAPTER 15:	Be Kind	36
CHAPTER 16:	Stab the Lab	37
CHAPTER 17:	Memory Test	38
CHAPTER 18:	Old Records	40
CHAPTER 19:	Bystanders	42
CHAPTER 20:	Gossip	43
CHAPTER 21:	Tests and More Tests	44

CHAPTER 22:	Diagnosis: Yours or Mine?	46
CHAPTER 23:	Criticizing the Previous Doctor	48
CHAPTER 24:	Minor Irritants, Loss of Focus	49
CHAPTER 25:	Emotional Blackmail, Warranty	50
CHAPTER 26:	Medical Jargon and Acronym	51
CHAPTER 27:	Medicine Dosage	54
CHAPTER 28:	Walking-in	57
CHAPTER 29:	Allergy	59
CHAPTER 30:	Fake News	60

SECTION 3: TO-DO LIST

CHAPTER 31:	Dress	65
CHAPTER 32:	How to Select a Specialist	68
CHAPTER 33:	Second Opinion	69
CHAPTER 34:	Tools to Carry	70

Index 71

Section 1

Two Way Traffic

CHAPTER 1: The Science

Compared to our ancestors, the Apes, we humans have attained a much longer life span (Chimpanzee 39 years, Bonobos 40 years) with an average global human life expectancy of 73.5 years at birth. But the main contrast is that while an ape's life expectancy has remained static, for us, it has galloped from 53 years in 1920, by a 20-year bonus, to 73 years by 2020. This increase is attributed to better living standards (better nutrition, improved hygiene, safe abode) reduction of infections and infestations (vaccines, antibiotics), better management of environment (flood, famine), and conflict reduction (war). The modern medical wonders like angioplasty, bypass surgery, or organ transplant have not added years to life but given us better *quality* life.

The main evolutionary change that came in as we lost our ancestral tail and fur was the development of language and a complex signaling system at the cellular level.

Evolution of language was indeed a game changer because it brought about a different level of communication beyond simple call for sex, an alarm for help, or a warning of a predator attack. Transfer of knowledge and skillset to others meant that learning was easily shared and the potential for excelling on the baseline skill was exponential.

At the cellular level, signaling systems evolved in a complex way so that internal cellular metabolism could be linked to the external environment in a much more sensitive manner. Humans could not just reshape their external environment like warming cars and cooling homes but alter cellular biology to survive extremes of Kalahari heat or the Siberian cold.

Such a sensitive system also meant that even in a comfortable room, we secrete more adrenalin watching a horror movie or oxytocin and dopamine when cuddled by our loved ones.

Many people believe that modern medicine has given us longer life. Galileo Galilei died in 1642 in Italy at the age of 77 years, Isaac Newton in 1727 in London at the age of 84, and Michelangelo in Rome in 1564 at the age of 88, much before many of modern medical marvels were invented. Modern medicine has *prevented* early death and certainly *improved quality of life*. We jog and play after a triple-vessel bypass surgery, we swim after a femur fracture and a hip replacement, and we check into a transatlantic flight after a heart transplant done for a failing heart that would have otherwise kept us tethered to oxygen in the intensive coronary care unit (ICCU).

So, the point is, we see our doctor to make sure that everything is fine; if not, he suggests remedies that let us enjoy the quality of life and freedom we so dearly enjoy.

In a study published in 2020, analysis of data from 30,933 cancer patients over a period of 14 years follow-up, the mortality (death rate) among those classified as "unhappy most of the time" versus those who were "happy most of the time", the unhappy group had a 78% higher hazard ratio of death. Happy people live longer. The first infusion of happiness or unhappiness from an ailment comes from your doctor when he discovers a disease. A disease with a death rate of 50% also has a survival rate of 50%.

CHAPTER 2: Setting the Stage

Death sentence—importance of those 5 minutes

Death sentences are usually read out by a serious-looking, bespeckled judge in a court room, filled with men in black robe, ending up with a thud of a hammer and a statement that the court is adjourned. All of us have seen this happen an umpteen number of times, in Netflix shows. But in real life, most death sentences are delivered by a man in a white coat, sitting on the other side of a working table, in a green room with a strong stench of disinfectant. The back-lit scan report is stuck up as a proof of your crime.

Take away the serial killers and mass murderers, and the rest of us would get the worst news of our lives during a routine consultation with our physician. Yes, most of us. And also the news about yourself or the people you love and care.

Good news is also transacted, here—telling you that you do not have cancer, or your cancer is cured, or that you are pregnant. But those are just stuff that is usual, right? The doctor just told you that you are not abnormal, at least for now. Never do you come out of a doctor's consultation with a news that you have won a lottery, gifted a Lamborghini, or found a girl of your dreams.

"Multiple metastatic shadows in the lungs and liver in the PET scan" in plain English language translates to a death sentence in about 12 months at the max, of which half of the time is spent in hospital bed, being pushed inside a dark suffocating tunnel of a whirring scanner, or let of women in white armed with a sharp needle and a professional smile asking you not to worry.

"Angiogram showing critical left-main with diffuse poorly graftable triple vessel disease, with gross LV dysfunction" means the only option left is to cut open your chest and rework the plumbing, and still you might need a wheelchair for the rest of your life.

Even a routine fever might turn out to be a dreadful "pancytopenia" or a diarrhea to a nuisance called "ulcerative colitis" needing lifelong treatment. These verdicts change your life.

Accepted, that as a patient, all that we can do is walk out depressed, but an early diagnosis, much before the cancer has spread, or the block in the heart has become nonsalvageable, we have a better chance of cure. Now, most of us, patients, would have seen our physician for a different purpose and the illness might not have been picked up. It is not that your doctor is not good enough but how well and how intelligently you presented your case to him. Those nonsignificant vague complaints that you have, from "gas" "dyspepsia" to jaw pain, might look trivial to you but ring an alarm bell to your physician's mind.

With today's array of ultraslice scanners to 3D imaging, does it matter as to how a patient presents to the physician? Well unfortunately, it does.

A patient with chest pain suggestive of a cardiac disease has a specific way of presenting itself, heavy, diffuse, a feeling of being unwell, restricting activities (angina). Your description of the discomfort rings an alarm bell in the mind of the physician, letting him check you out. Interestingly, in angina, the ECG, echocardiogram, and even the angiogram (especially in women) may be normal. If you do not tell the doctor about your symptoms, it is unlikely that your angina will ever be diagnosed and treated.

Your doctor is busy, not just trying to relieve your symptoms or trying to see if any of your symptoms raise a red flag for more workup, but a host of boring administration work, including documentation, investigation, insurance forms, and billing needs to be done in the background.

Think of it, most of us would see a doctor with either fever, headache, tiredness, or chest or stomach pain. To the doctor, who sees hundreds of such patients, majority turns out to be nothing. A paracetamol here and an antibiotic there with a cough syrup and an antacid would do the job. But when it does not work or it presents with an odd symptom, the doctor tends to sit up. The challenge is more in India because your doctor would be seeing, on an average, 10 times more patients compared to a US physician. Also, Indian patients are fascinated by medical degrees, and doctors enjoy flaunting them in dozens, covering every single alphabet in the dictionary. There are patients who keep on seeing their gastroenterologist with stomach pain which is actually cardiac, and I continue to treat, possible unnecessarily, unrelated medical problems since their ECG shows some variation. Had these patients seen a good general physician first, a lot of trouble could have been avoided. Decluttering the health system is extremely important, but we are not talking about it now.

If I asked you to recall what you think to be the most important milestones of Steve Jobs life, you would perhaps list the incorporation of Apple in 1977, introduction of iPod in 2001, iPhone debut in 2007, or his famous Stanford commencement speech in 2005. But asked the same question, Steve Jobs himself would say, it was that day in 2004, when during a routine health check-up his doctor detected the presence of a pathology in his pancreatic gland, which finally turned out to be pancreatic cancer. A life-changing diagnosis.

iPhone or iPad might have changed the life of many of us, but for Jobs himself it was the diagnosis that changed his own life course.

Life-changing events can happen by accident just about anywhere—a mall store might catch fire, a road trip end up in a car crash, or a routine flight fall off the sky—but these are rare accidents. They regularly scroll-crawl along the x-axis of TV screen but they are distinctly rare. But a doctor's office and hospital are places where life-changing events take place as a routine, almost by *design*. We are born and eventually die in hospitals. Today, you actually need a lot of luck to die peacefully at home. The society, your family, friends, and neighborhood would make sure that you are not allowed to pass away peacefully at home. Most major illnesses are diagnosed here, in the hospital. The shadow in the X-ray or the mass in the scan might turn out to be a highly invasive cancer or a mere false alarm, life changing either way.

Surprisingly, a medical checkup is traditionally never looked upon as a "life-changing" encounter. We routinely wish people a safe flight but not a good luck as they go to meet their doctor.

The doctor listens to our complaints, examines us, and suggests tests, scans, and may be a biopsy. The radiologist looks at the scans, the pathologist at the cells under a microscope, and a diagnosis emerges. If the cells under the microscope look normal, you would go back home whistling; if the pathologist found some abnormal cells, you may end up on the operating table and end up losing a limb or a breast.

Today, studies after studies have shown that more and more young, highly talented, extremely skilled doctors, interventional cardiologists, surgeons, anesthetists, and critical care specialists are heading for a *burnout* (a term indicating that they would become medically useless) and many are already neck deep into it. It is also known that the more stressed the doctor is, the more likely he is going for a burnout at Godspeed. The stressed doctor is likely to commit more professional mistakes in their decisions, which might be just a piece of mistake for him but may cost you your life.

Patients ask doctors as to what are "my chances of getting cured". A medical answer of 80% would appease him, but neither the patient nor the doctor knows if he belonged to the good 80% or the bad 20%. Medical statistics is good for a population and a group, but tells nothing about an individual's response to a treatment. So after discussing all the options, when you doctors say, "I think chemotherapy is better than surgery for you", he is trying to match the statistics with his experience of your kind of cases that he has seen and make a logical conclusion. So that means it is extremely important that he does it for you in a stable state of mind, by applying all his cognitive energy. An irritated doctor, upset by a silliest reason, and thus making a different judgment (not wrong or right but the best for you) could change the course of your life. It is important that he is smiling because a smiling "cool" doctor is more likely to take a correct decision for you.

Human body looks so beautiful and proportionate outside but was designed to have no user-serviceable parts, which explains for the lack of screws and fasteners. The only way doctors can go inside is to cut it open or sometimes entering through natural ports or punctures. When spliced open, it does not look good at all. A brown-colored heart with yellow fats as fillers, a pair of soggy wet lungs, coils of slippery intestine filled with gooey material, oozing blood and lymph, even the best surgical fields are not a nice visual to watch, worse than the tangled wires and chipset of a PC.

Agreed that doctors are professionals, and most excel in what they do, catching the disease by its tail, they throw away the serpentine curse swiftly before it can use its fangs on us.

Doctors deal with torn arms, wounded torso, bleeding nose, broken bones, and dilated heart. They watch people sob in pain, cry of loss, stunned by sorrow, suffer from shock and disbelief of tragedy, and often are duty bound to watch people die. Most part of the day, they have to face and talk to people who are facing the darkest moments of their life and that is not funny. It is not humanly possible to move quickly from a dying patient, detach yourself emotionally, and smile and laugh a few minutes later because the next patient has told him something funny.

If you thought that medical school toughens a doctor, you are right and wrong. Right because we do not faint at the sight of blood or vomit at the smell of rotten body parts, but most would react to their kids' school-day drama performance or their mom's disability with the same degree of enthusiasm and desperation like anyone else. Watching people suffer day in and day out takes its toll on anybody's mind.

Don't you want that at every stage of your illness, the doctor—the physician, the surgeon, the radiologist, the pathologist, and the anesthesiologist be not just the best in business but fully focused on your problem so that you do well? A stressed-out, angry radiologist, a dissatisfied pathologist, or a grumpy physician would be the last of your hospital bucket list.

As you would see reading further, an unhappy, stressed, grumpy doctor may not always make a correct diagnosis; even when he hits the bull's eye, he might not logically think of the best options available, or choose one which is right for you. But fortunately, these are rare.

But what is common is vital for you.

Once a diagnosis is made, it is easy to look into many of the options available. Search google for breast cancer and you would find millions of hits in a fraction of a second, from chemotherapy to diet therapy and nature therapy, from radiotherapy to immunotherapy and everything in between. Now, the next question is which of these is best for you. Biochemistry, histopathology, and even genetic testing narrow down the choice further. But still multiple options remain. That is where your physician's opinion counts. Not just an opinion but direction, decision and way forward.

Modern medicine teaches doctors on offering all available options to the patient, based on evidence-based medicine, and there are many. The philosophy is to let the *patient* choose the best option. This has become more important in the days of litigation, where the doctor's decision might be scrutinized under a magnifying glass later to detect flaws in his diagnosis and treatment. But medicine is about taking chances too. The first recipient of penicillin or insulin never imagined that they are the first lucky ones to receive a life-changing therapy. The first recipient of pacemaker, Arne Larsson, aged 43 years, did not think that he would receive 26 times changes of the pulse generator (those days pacemakers lasted for few years) but subsequently outlive the engineer who devised it and the doctor who implanted it. He died in 2002 at 86 years of age. But many others who received such trial "*experimental*" therapy, hoping to get a miracle cure, did not live long enough to tell their stories of failure.

CHAPTER 3

Inside the Doctor's Mind

Patients go to a doctor mostly with a complaint, a trouble that is called *symptom*. Derived from Greek word *"Sumpipto"* meaning "I fall", symptoms started to mean *any discomfort that patient felt*, from *severe headache* to a *numb toe*, from *hacking cough* to *chronic constipation*, and everything in between that troubled a patient. In olden days, what the patient wanted was to get relief from his symptoms. The same applies for most of us today too.

Then came the concept of disease, a heart attack, a gastric ulcer, a rib fracture, or a pneumonia that could all cause a chest pain but needed different treatment. It was not enough to relieve the pain but vital to treat the underlying pathology. So, from the concept of *symptom relief*, we graduated to *disease cure*. The concept was so disruptive that doctors started giving minimum importance to symptom relief. Symptomatic treatment is considered an inferior therapy where the doctor is yet to grasp a proper diagnosis.

A common complaint like fever or chest pain can come because of hundreds of different diseases. A fever could turn out to be a simple viral fever or a complicated pneumonia or meningitis. A chest pain could be a massive heart attack or just dyspepsia. A thyroid disease or a lymphoma (a type of cancer) can start off with a symptom of fever.

The doctor takes a detailed history and orders screening tests to pick up any red flags of a serious disease, and once those are negative he gives symptomatic treatment. A simple paracetamol or a pantoprazole would take care of dyspepsia and viral fever. Only if it fails to give relief does the doctor ask for more detailed tests. There is hardly a way to suspect or a test to confirm an unusual infection or a complicated autoimmune/metabolic disease on day 1 of a fever.

ALGORITHM AND EPIDEMIOLOGY

Algorithm is derived from an Arabic word *"algorism"* which literally means *"reuniting broken parts"*. It was 780 AD. A kid was born to Musa in the town of Khwarizmi in Persia. He was named Abu. Abu turned out to be a genius, a polymath, who, among many other firsts, discovered the basics of algebra. Abu, son of *Musa*, from *Khwarizmi*—"Abu Abdullah Muhammad ibn Musa Al-Khwarizmi", wrote about the connecting link of Arabic numerals to Hindu methods of mathematics, which was later translated to Latin as *"Algoritmi de numero Indorum"*. Over time, a set of rules, which drive or guide anything to a logical conclusion, became known as "algorithm". From detecting a bug in a software to finding out the cause of fever in a child, algorithms set the rules as to how to go forward.

The idea looked brilliant, but there was another problem when applied to medicine.

The disease prevalence varied depending on locations. While the common cause of a persistent fever in south Africa is likely to be malaria, in western USA it is Rocky Mountain Spotted Fever or West Nile Virus, while in Japan it could be Japanese Tick Fever. Post 2019, COVID-19 pandemic changed all that. This highlights the importance of knowing what disease is prevalent in the location that a doctor practices. The science of distribution of disease is called epidemiology.

Epidemiology is a modifier of the medical diagnostic algorithm locally.

HEURISTICS

Heuristics is a shortcut, used by the human mind in an emergency.

A small kid walking across a road is apparently unaware of an approaching truck. A passer-by dashes across and picks up the child right on time, seconds before the truck passes. Such deeds do not leave you time to think. It is some kind of complex reflex that humans have developed, reserved only for emergencies. In a medical emergency, sometimes there is no time to think. The physician acts reflexively, a reflex developed and honed over years of practice, which could sometimes turn out to be wrong too.

CHAPTER 4
Specialization and Loss of Family Physician

If the color pink describes the best of health; in my childhood, I was hovering between shades of grey; febrile fits, tons of tonsillitis, yearly earache, and blight appetite. The only bright patch for my parents to look forward to was our family doctor. He was a tall, fair, heavily built gentleman sporting a "breaking-news" smile and carrying a "sniffer-dog-baiting" brown bag; he was the "one-stop shop" for all medical and sometimes nonmedical problems.

No one enquired about his medical degree, doubted his diagnosis, or queried about potential side effects of the medicine that he dispensed through his "compounder", but almost everyone got relieved of their symptoms.

"What's a compounder? Sounds like a cool *android app*", commented my son, a final year medical student, who prereads my manuscripts.

"Well it's a fusion of a secretary, a nurse, a pharmacist and PR manager, all rolled into one single package. I believe he compounded the treatment effect of the doctor".

With no cellphone notifications to distract him, the doctor would attentively listen to complaints, examine patients, holding his long dark stethoscope with utmost respect, prescribe medicines, and give injections, while the compounder prepared the "soap-water" tasting mixture.

From headache to leg cramps, dyspepsia to back pain, and joints stiffened by arthritis or loosened during football, he had remedy for everything. Symptom relief was all that patients sought from their doctors, and they got it, most of the time.

Three things happened that made the "all-in-one doctor" (aka family doctor) and his compounder to disappear in the process of social evolution.

The first medical professionals understood that most symptoms reflect an underlying disease; treating just the symptom is not enough. Subsidence of chest pain or stomach cramp or a headache does not do much good in the long run but clearing the block in the heart, which led to chest pain, or removal of the gall stone or brain tumor does.

The second change came in when medicine embraced "technology" in a big way, from complex biochemistry to scanning, from needle biopsy to endoscopy, CT, PET, MRI; the boundless progress of diagnostic science impressed everyone, and the physician was no exception. All that the doctor now had to do was to know which test to order for which disease, and the laboratory would test, scan, or image and send back the diagnosis, with an accuracy far exceeding the clinician's physical sense. Interpret the disease and the doctor's job is done. A 3-minute listening could not fight the glamour of a 3-million-dollar MRI.

The third tsunami was data archiving; started initially to refer to the individual patient's old record to compare and decide progression of disease, it soon expanded to the assessment of treatment benefit of the populations at large (epidemiological data) like efficacy of vaccinations and antibiotics. And then, data became important for legal purposes as people wanted doctors to explain and justify their action and failures, in the court of law.

Introduction of computers made it possible to store megabytes of data available for analysis, which quickly moved up in scale to gigabytes and petabytes.

Today, the doctor is busy putting your data in his system, ordering and interpreting the laboratory and imaging results and making sure that he remains in his consultation room in white coat, most of the time, rather than standing in the witness box in the company of black robes.

The patient came with chest pain; all tests including angiogram turned out to be normal.

"So you have no problem at all", I said, showing off one of my best smiles.

"But doctor my pain is still there".

I refer him to general medicine, gastroenterologist, neurologist, and if needed psychiatrist.

From my point of view as a cardiologist, he has no cardiac problems; it is just nothing.

A nuisance of sorts to me.

But for him, it still hurts.

His confused look reminded me of the customer standing in front of the long shelf in the supermarket with hundreds of brands and no one to help him choose.

May be, we need the family doctor back, with an upgraded, *Java* enabled "compounder".

CHAPTER 5
Accidents and Family Reunion: India is Different

Crash landings are always bad and horrific, but timing can still make a huge difference on the overall outcome.

On a chilly morning on January 15, 2009, captain Chesley Burnett Sullenberger "sully" crash landed US Airways flight 1549 on the freezing waters of Hudson river. With both engines down, landing safely was a huge challenge; his timely decision made sure that no one lost their life. Aviation specialists worldwide agree that his glide timing was perfect.
Timing is what matters.

This was another crash landing, perfectly timed.

She was an 85-year-old lady, salt-pepper hair, sand-dune forehead, a toothless fairy. It turned out later that she too had chosen the timing of her crash fairly well, just a day prior to a long weekend in the United States and a day after the school closure holidays in Dubai.

This was one place in hospital where my white coat was clearly out of place. The large air-conditioned "suite" room was located in the hospital's exclusive deluxe floor, meant for those who earned their salary in dirhams or dollars. As I entered the room, the atmosphere clearly reflected a festive mood—two kids were trying to play with toy cars, a bored teenager was fiddling with a smartphone, three young men presumably "*co-brothers*" with thick gold bracelets laughing loudly sharing a joke between them, and two ladies seriously scrutinizing new jewelry style of a third subject.

The epicenter of the whole circus, an elderly *ammumma* (grandmother), was dozing on the hospital cot, with a sandbag of 5 kg hung from her fractured right leg; she looked so much out of place.

On the sides were multiple large boxes and cartons with Chinese and Arabic labels; the airline tags confirming that the concerned relatives had hurriedly left home to scramble on the board of an aircraft and rushed to the hospital straight from the arrival lounge.

"Oh the doctor is here", a murmur breaks out.

CHAPTER 5: Accidents and Family Reunion: India is Different

The jokes stop, the precious-metal investigation paused, the teenager sits erect, and the kids continue their business on the race track.

"So doctor, at what time are you contemplating surgery? Between 10 and 11 AM is a good time", one *cobra* comments.

I am just a cardiology doctor; I am here to clear her for surgical fitness. "The orthopedic doctor will tell you the exact time".

"Oh ok doctor, thank you".

I could feel the attention level coming down. It is like eagerly waiting for the superstar; instead, it turns out to be the makeup man.

I examine the lady.

She had a fracture of the hip, a common fracture that elderly people sustain on fall. It needs a hip-replacement surgery. The ECG shows a subtle sign of ischemia, her pulse is irregular, hemoglobin is low, and the creatinine is little high.

As I slowly try to talk about the problems, I hear a familiar sigh.

"We know that she has problems; these come up with age. But doctor I am in Texas, and I have to go back to the US next Thursday latest; my co-brother here has an assignment at Dubai. We were *lucky* that the fall happened a day before the long weekend; so I could immediately get a ticket for all of us. My co-brother at Dubai had a problem of getting leave, but he too managed. If possible, please see that the surgery is not delayed".

"I shall talk to the orthopedic", I announce meekly, sounding like an airline employee announcing a possible flight delay and end up in a cancellation.

"Doctor, we normally come home at least once a year to see *ammumma*, but at different times. After 10 long years, we are all here together, at the same time. Our kids are so excited; you see".

I could see.

The surgery proceeded well. She was shifted back after a day's stay in the intensive coronary care unit (ICCU). The bystanders thanked me for all the help.

It was a week past her surgery and physiotherapy; *ammumma* was ready to go home. I went for the routine rounds. The room was deserted except for some empty boxes and chocolate wrappers. A "bored" elderly lady announced, "I am the home nurse; sirs have all gone back and told me to take care. They call me every other day and get updated".

An optimally timed crash in an Indian home can cause a turmoil in the Texas, disruption in Dubai, and, of course, a long-awaited picnic of people, gathering at God's own country.

The approach to an illness is different depending on whether or not you are educated and imbibe eastern or western culture. In East, as we age, we tend to depend on our younger generation for help and support. A three-generation Indian family is a perfect example of this philosophy. While the grandparents take care of the grandchildren, the parents work and earn for their education. The elder grandparents' needs are taken care of by the family. With a poor health insurance coverage, this system holds good, but import of western culture with an intense importance on privacy and independence has put enormous pressure on the system. Now the elderly population has to go out and take care of themselves. Being nonjudgmental about the merits and demerits of the conservative, safety-first eastern culture, compared to the intense privacy-driven attitude of the west, the Indian health system is at crossroads.

CHAPTER 6

More Insight: East versus West

"Daughter from California" syndrome is a phrase used in medical profession to describe a situation in which a hitherto disengaged relative challenges the care a dying elderly patient is being given, or insists that the medical team pursue aggressive measures to prolong the patient's life—*Wikipedia*.

With a large number of software engineers migrating to the Silicon Valley the "daughter from California" syndrome has reached the Indian shores. Frantic calls from abroad are fueled by concerns for their parents' health, a very low rating of the health care facility available in India, the guilt of being unable to be physically present with the family, and the western metrics of assessment of health. Comments like "why not heart transplant" and "connected to life-support system" are used casually without understanding the pain, the quality of life, and the economic consequences of a disease and its treatment.

Most "East" versus "West" debate about healthcare ends up as a fight between traditional data-scant "Ayurvedic" medical practice of the "East" versus the evidence-based, robust, "Modern" medicine of the "West". But there is a huge unappreciated cultural and philosophic chasm between "East" and "West".

▪ AGING GRACEFULLY IN DIFFERENT WAYS

— ♦ ♦ ♦ —

Case 1

"You know what sir? The doctors in the other hospital told us that they wanted to do a *bypass* surgery for our '83-year-old' mother. We don't want her to undergo complicated medical procedure unless there is a crisis. We understand that from the medical point of view, a *bypass* may be necessary, but she is 83 years and intolerant *even* to an injection pain. Moreover, presently she has no chest pain, and continues to do her daily *pooja* (religious rituals). Since the doctors there were unhappy with us for refusing surgery, we got her discharged and brought her to you for a consultation. We are happy as long as she is comfortable, but we can't see our mother suffer from complicated surgical procedure even if it extends her life by few years. We would wish to take her home and care for her. Our mother means everything to us sir".

The man in *dhoti and kurta* (traditional Indian attire) was emotional.

"The kids at home, my son and daughter, are eagerly waiting for their grandmother to come home and tell them stories", the man was almost in tears.

"Sir, one more request, please *don't tell her* that there are severe blocks in her heart. *We want her to live worry-free*, whatever is left of her life".

"What is *her* take on bypass?", I ask.

"She says she will follow whatever we decide best for her".

―◆◆◆―

Case 2

"You know doc, the doctor in the other hospital said that my dad was too old for an angiography and bypass surgery; too old! Can you imagine; in this era of evidence-based medicine, a doctor is refusing treatment on the basis of his age? I was truly upset. I don't really know what kind of medical practice goes around in India. Yes, I agree, he is 87; but how can a doctor decide on a treatment based on age? I work as software specialist in the California. I was told that you are academically very bright and trained in the US. And that's why we are here".

The lady in skinny jeans, clutching an oversized I-phone, talking in an American accent was truly concerned. She did not want to deny any effective treatment to her father.

"And doc, please tell my father in details what you make out of his illness; the procedures you plan; the complication expected – everything. *He should know it after all*".

Despite opposing views, I think *both* the conservative "East" and the aggressive "West" are *right*, in their own perspective, and one need not be judged by the other.

The intense desire of right of independence and the sensitivity to individual privacy inculcated in the western culture come at a cost of loneliness in an advanced age, especially with the demise of a partner. The ingrained right to choose options *ourselves*, one of the tenets on which modern medical ethics is built up, is *undeniably robust*. It also explains as to why doctors are so upset when people choose options that are against "evidence-based medicine" and when someone else makes a choice on behalf of the patient. We feel, justifiably so, that it is our duty to let the patient know every bit of what we know about his illness.

We may be right, but it is not wrong for any *culturally divergent group to reject our notion.*

The aggressiveness of medical therapy as age advances, as well as the patient and family participation in decision-making, depends on our upbringing and education. It holds true for the patients and the doctors alike.

The practice of medicine should be nonjudgmental and meant ultimately to make our patients happy. From tablets to injections, from physiotherapy to angioplasty, the foremost intention of every medical therapy is to make the patient comfortable.

It doesn't really matter if it is eastern "philosophy" of *senescence* or western "evidence-based" *independence*.

CHAPTER 7
Kerb-side Consult: Right or Wrong?

In the morning, between newspaper and coffee, I chose reading the newspaper and let my wife have the pleasure of making coffee. Surely I miss out the misty, smoky, hill-station-like atmosphere of the kitchen, but you cannot have the best of everything. The deal is clear. Once she gives me the hot coffee, within the next 2 hours I hand over the cold newspaper in return; that works fine for me.

My wife is an expert in nutrition and believes in evidence-based science, and that is why two thin arrowroot biscuits come bundled with the coffee, to make sure that neither of my family traits of diabetes and hair loss affects me.

"The maid's husband's brother's cholesterol report is here", she points out to the neatly folded paper under the saucer.

"I think the cholesterol is high. Why don't you write some medicines?", my wife asked.

Over the years, I have learnt that a friendly suggestion from the admin is to be always taken as orders.

I am reminded of the article that recently appeared in the leading medical journal "Lancet" on "Stop kerb-side consultation" advising doctors not to write a prescription unless they thoroughly examine a patient and is aware about their past medical details. "The risk involved in casual consultation is unacceptable", it commented.

Let us say you meet your architect during the morning walk, your plumber in the fish market, or the advocate in the shopping mall. Would you think it appropriate to ask the architect whether you can have the kitchen relocated, the plumber about the leaky faucet, or the advocate on his legal advice on your impending divorce?

But for a doctor, it is different.

"Hello uncle, how are you" is mostly answered with "I have some 'gas' problem; can you tell me some good medicines", followed by a statement like "your auntie is worrying type and thinks that gas trouble may actually be some heart problem, so I thought you are the *best person* to ask".

"But the narrow gap between the shelfs of the margin-free market is not just the *best place*.....", but social etiquette makes me keep quiet.

CHAPTER 7: Kerb-side Consult: Right or Wrong?

Look at a water-filled beaker by passing an oblique ray of light, and you see randomly moving particles. Physics students call it "Brownian movement", chaos in simple terms. But to a doctor, the real chaos is an overcrowded medical outpatient department. Suffering patients, irate bystanders, angry nurses, hypothyroid secretaries, and expressionless doctors make a perfect combination of chaos.

As I am trying to concentrate on the lub-dup with the stethoscope on his chest, the patient takes out a paper from his pant pocket.

"Reports", he smiles.

I feel irritated but glance at the report.

"Your blood sugar is too high", I say.

"That's actually my *wife's* sugar report, you had asked me to bring it when I came to see you".

I am stumped.

A middle-aged man and an elderly lady compete with each other to hand me their blood report and X-ray. I try to replay my memory at double speed to play back as to why did I order them.

"Do you have my old prescription?"

"No, doctor, but you only asked me to do all these tests 7 days back".

In the last 1 week, I had seen 50 patients a day with 50 different problems. And I have grown 1 week older; don't you know that with age, memory deteriorates? Silence is golden.

After examining token number 43, an elderly lady, I notice that the bystander, a young man in his 20s, has a swollen neck.

"Do you have thyroid complaints?"

"No sir".

I called him aside and examined his neck.

It was an unusually hard thyroid nodule; I had a strong suspicion that it is not a good disease.

I asked him to consult the surgeon.

"No, not next week, not tomorrow. Today". I insisted.

The surgeon confirmed the diagnosis as papillary carcinoma, a type of thyroid cancer. Three days later, he had a total thyroid gland-removal surgery. That was 5 years ago; he still comes with his mother for follow-up.

The young girl standing by the side of the grandmother looked normal except for a little fidgety nature, which many 10-year-old girls have. But this was different. It looked like a case of chorea, a movement disorder that affects kids with rheumatic fever. A referral to the neurologist confirmed the unusual disease and cured it.

In the chaos-prone health system in India, kerb-side consultation is indispensable, as indispensable as the "auto rickshaw" and "mango pickles".

This all highlights the understanding that practice of medicine is so different between the conservative east and the maverick west.

CHAPTER 8: Investigations, and More

A doctor tries his best to arrive at a provisional diagnosis, when he first sees a patient. So, the fever with no red flag on day 1 (most will not have one) is treated as a viral fever with a simple paracetamol tablet, topped with an antihistaminic, if you have a clogged nose or a sore throat. Does he try to rule out complex cancers (lymphoma) or a brain abscess on day 1? Certainly no. That is not how a medical algorithm works. If there is any red flag like unusual headache or swollen glands, it is different, but otherwise no.

He has no problem in asking for a brain scan and elaborate blood checks for the child, on day 1 itself, but it is a wastage of resources and time; moreover, the results might turn out to be confusing, thus ending up in more tests.

But if a doctor is asked, "why don't you do more tests", he would take the easy way out and order all possible investigations.

Forcing your doctor to overinvestigate not only burdens the system but could confuse the doctor and might end up in a botched treatment.

CHAPTER 9
Opinion, Option, or Direction

Even after 3 decades of medical practice, I often wonder as to what could be the best form of therapy for a person with multiple blocks—medicine, angioplasty or bypass surgery. Obviously, my data-spewing lecture of evidence-based advise is going to further confuse the patient. It is like the ordinary British citizen overwhelmingly choosing Brexit, mostly not clearly knowing what it is.

So what you want from your doctor is to choose the therapy that is *right* for you. A surgery that is curable for someone maybe too risky for you. A medicine that is magical for the white Caucasian may not work for the brown Asian or the black African.

The final question we all ask is, "doctor, tell me what you think is best for me". Or "what would you choose if it was your mom?"

So we, you, me everyone, need a clear-thinking doctor who would think about us as his own family and give us a direction that he feels is appropriate just for me. It is not the options that the patient wants but a right direction from those confusing options. A 20% risk of a procedure does not make sense because you could fall in the good 80% or the unfortunate 20%. You want your doctor to use his experience and expertise to tell you his gut feeling of what is best for you.

Take it from me, today most doctors would list out all the available options for you with the available statistics of possible outcome and ask *you to choose the one you feel the best for you*, because that is the *safest legal bet* for the doctor. That way, you (or your family) can never blame the doctor for not discussing a particular option. Only if the doctor considers you close enough would he commit to one option, telling you that option A is better than option B for you. Not the data, but what he makes out of the data that is *best for you*. And that is the very reason you have gone to him.

As long as the doctor sees the patient as his client with a potential to sue him at the slightest mistake, it will not happen. Only if the patient and the doctor join as a team, looking and tackling the problem together, it will turn out right.

Sitting on the opposite side of the table, passing a verdict will no longer be tenable in the future. The doctor and the patient have to sit on the same side of the table and face disease.

It is only then that the doctor's option will become an opinion; he will choose the best for you, so that you do not need to google search and get puzzled with a billion of options.

CHAPTER 10: Doctor Relative

Let us presume that you have a complex cardiac issue, and you have three different opinions from three different cardiologists. Your brother is a cardiologist himself. You talk to him. He asks you to go for an angioplasty and not bypass surgery or medical treatment. All the three eminent doctors had given you *options* and opinion from their perspective. But your brother would have given you a *direction* thinking about your perspective as his own. So, it is obvious that you would follow him. What if every time an opinion is given, the doctor tells you about the *options* as well as which of these he feels is best for you; that is *direction*. Ten years down the line, if your angioplasty fails, you will not question your brother for a wrong decision, because you know that you have weighed all options and decided to choose the one best for you, in the best of everyone's interest. That is because you have total faith on your brother, who *knows the evidence* and has the relationship to *show you the right direction*. That is what you want out of your doctor during those 5 minutes.

This can happen only of the doctor believes that you will not counterquestion him regarding his motive for that particular opinion. I can list out all the options available to you, but I would point to the *best direction that I feel is best for you* only if I am under no obligation or legal binding to do so.

Your doctor should feel free and confidant to tell you about all the options and point out the one that he thinks is best for you. If he feels that it is best to take a second opinion, he should feel free to tell you that. In case of half of extremely complicated cases I see, I discuss with the patient the need for another opinion. Most patients answer, "Okay doctor if you feel like I will take a second opinion but I would go by your final opinion".

If the doctor and patients are sitting on the same side of the table, handhold and face the disease together, it would forge the best partnership and ensure the best possible outcome.

Section 2

Real Life

CHAPTER 11

Timing is Everything

---♦♦♦---

"Doctor?"

"Yes"

"Doctor, what's your consultation time at home?"

"6 pm till 8 pm".

"Thanks. In that case shall I come by 8:15; *by then you would be free I think*".

---♦♦♦---

Most people think that doctors are doctors 24/7/365 and they are right. The same applies for an architect, an engineer, and a policeman. But all such 24/7 services are run by a system, not one individual. Doctors have a consultation schedule and it would be the best to follow it, unless it is an emergency. While the patient's definition of emergency could be an irritating complaint (symptom) like a pain, to the doctor an acute emergency would be a catastrophic cardiac or a neurologic disease. In case of an emergency, it is always advisable to get in touch with a system (emergency room) rather than calling up your doctor, who might underestimate your problem. Most people presume that asking the doctor about the reason for his headache, or a remedy for stomach upset, or discussing about their cholesterol report is a small talk, is okay, and is not something official. Try asking your architect about the door's location of your upcoming home or the lawyer about the legal validity of a court document during an accidental meeting as you take a stroll in the park.

Suppose you meet a doctor during a casual chat and he suggests a tablet for you, and that tablet results in a severe side effect; would you not feel bad? By the way, if you are wondering as to why should a doctor write a medicine with such side effects at all, there is no single pill without a side effect except just one. It is called placebo.

The common paracetamol tablet that we gulp without a second thought has a long list of complications including rare and fatal liver failure.

Sixty minutes before the flight, the check-in closes and the gates shut 30 minutes before the flight, whether or not you board the flight. So is the train, the post office, or the bank. Do make sure that you are on your appointed time, perhaps a little before to consult your doctor. You reach the doctor's clinic to see your token number fading, before being replaced by the next number; you run up to his door, argue with the nurse, give a cold look at the patients with a token next to you, and manage to jostle in; it is fine. But do you realize that your heart rate is likely to be fast and BP high which might end up in your doctor assessing you wrongly and prescribing unnecessary medicines?

"The doctor will be little late, he is stuck in an emergency".

"The departure time is rescheduled because of a technical problem".

"Unable to connect to internet in view of heavy internet traffic, please try later".

All of this are unbelievable, made up.

But yes, we do not want to board a faulty aircraft or ask the doctor stop doing an emergency angioplasty to a critical patient, but we hate to wait. Exactly like a pilot who would refuse to fly an aircraft that is 99% okay, the doctor cannot leave an emergency patient, even at the cost of inconvenience to dozens of cursing patients and relatives waiting with an appointment booked weeks earlier. And most busy doctors have to attend emergencies, frequently.

This is what the doctor is used to hearing:

"Doctor I reached your OPD at 10, and waiting for 2 long hours now".

This is what he does not tell you.

"I reached at 6 because I had an emergency call, and didn't even get a chance to go back home or shower, but yes I know that doesn't matter to you".

CHAPTER 12

Gas

Shapeless, colorless, and invisible, the most intriguing state of matter is "gas". Cocooned in steel cylinders in a hospital as "oxygen", it can save hundreds of lives; released in atmosphere in 1984 as "methyl isocyanate", it wiped out 5,000 lives overnight in Bhopal. Not surprising that it derives its name from Greek word *"Khaos"* transformed to Dutch *"chaos"* (random movement)—and finally *"gas".*

Robert Boyle in 1662, Jacques Charles in 1784, and later Avogadro tried their best to clarify the physical behavior of gas relating to volume, pressure, temperature, and molecular mass, but they could not anticipate or guess its more important "sociobiological" effects on the medical diagnostic dilemma in the years to come.

The molecular physics of "gas" met the cellular biology for the first time in 1842 when Dr Crawford Long used "ether" vapor to numb surgical pain at Massachusetts General Hospital at Boston. Public realization that the technique was safe came in for the first time when *anesthetic gas* was used for Queen Victoria's "painless" childbirth in 1853.

The "gas" finally reached the brain.

— ♦ ♦ ♦ —

"But you had this chest discomfort for the last 3 days, why didn't you come to the hospital earlier?"

The patient and his family could sense the frustration in my tone. He was a teacher in a college teaching commerce. His ECG showed a massive heart attack that was at least 72 hours old. Delay in presentation tends to worsen the outcome of a heart attack substantially, even if the block was cleared.

"Doctor, I thought that it was gas that has come up to my chest."

"He gets such symptoms when he takes *sambar*", added his wife. "Do you think we need to repeat the ECG to reconfirm?"

I could feel her problem in accepting the disease.

Despite Dan Brown's description of hidden viaducts and subterrain tunnels in various Italian cities, such an access of "gas" traveling from stomach to chest is still unknown to the medical community.

Most Indian doctors are intrigued by the diverse manifestations of "gas" which was never taught to them in medical school; from heart attack to breathing trouble, from sleeplessness to muscle cramps, disc prolapse to appendicitis, many of these unrelated diseases are attributed to gas. Every friendly neighbor is ready with his explanation of gas and offer his magical remedy, which the patient cannot refuse.

Many bad diseases can have a bloating sensation of the abdomen and belching, but self-labeling everything as gas and delaying diagnosis and treatment is sometimes dangerous.

We had a patient of cerebral hemorrhage presenting with headache which the patient attributed to "potato-induced" gas going to the head; for another lady, pulmonary embolism (lung clot) reminded her of "gas-in-the-lungs" resulting from eating tapioca. Despite a turbulent in-hospital course, both of them survived.

An American medical student who had spent some time with us mistook a patient's gas problem as nonavailability of car fuel (gasoline), but quickly assimilated the Indian philosophy of gas being the nidus of diagnostic confusion of many diseases.

Hundred years back, we would attribute all diseases to the curse of God. Unravelling the complexities and ambiguity of human biology has given us insights into many mysterious diseases. Early diagnosis promises a better outcome. Let us not blindly blame everything to gas and miss out or delay the diagnosis of a major malady.

Remember that it may not be just "laughing gas".

CHAPTER 13

Doc Scare

A busy day with two heart attack admissions in the morning, one patient on ventilator, I was already 1 hour behind schedule in the outpatient department (OPD).

Suddenly, my cell phone rang.

"Hello Doctor, I am your daughter's chemistry teacher".

"Good morning teacher, how are you"?

"I am just outside your OPD with my aunt who needs a checkup. Her token number is 38".

I looked at the display board, which showed no. 12. I could hear the irate shouts of impatient patients waiting since morning who were almost fed up. My daughter's chemistry mark flashed in front of me. The confidant, nice, friendly cardiologist in me started to lose his cool.

It is not just the inconvenience that counts. From politicians to policemen, from celebrities to businessmen, doctors get recommendations for an early appointment. It is not just queue jumping, but the whole system is disrupted, and the doctor and his team have to be apologetic to the rest of the OPD crowd waiting to see, who are intelligent enough to spot the queue jumpers but decent enough not to protest. The moment the doctor knows that the patient is special, the doctor is under stress and puts on all the defense armors to make sure that he does not miss anything. He is now more bothered about his missing something, rather than the patient's well-being. This increases the investigation bulk and the delay in treatment and overall creates a guarded approach to the problem.

It is very likely that in such a case he will lay out *all the options* available to the patients and their merits and demerits but *unlikely to point out to what he would do if he was the patient.* Options sans direction.

It is important to catch the attention of your doctor. It is important that he understands and recognizes your problem in a crowded OPD. It is also important that he is not scared enough to put on his protective mental armor. Let him tell you his direction, not the options of crossroads available to you.

CHAPTER 14: Teaching the Doctor

A lot of doctors get angry when a patient comes armed with a google search or checks the diagnosis online.

I happen to be the member of the four-member "Hypertension Council" of the Cardiological Society of India (CSI), the apex committee that charts out hypertension guidelines in India. I am also in the editorial board of half a dozen of journals.

Two contrasting cases prove the point I am aiming at.

—◆◆◆—

"Doctor did you know that there is a new 'plant-based' medicine that cures hypertension with just 5 doses; and, no side effects like allopathic medicines. I found out in Google yesterday?"

Clearly, I did not.

But I could get a fair idea of his IQ.

—◆◆◆—

One of my relatives called me over phone and sent me her medical details. She has lately developed hypertension and diabetes. She managed to check basic blood work from a local laboratory which was normal. I tweaked her medication dosage, again online. Two weeks later, she was still feeling fatigued, which we attributed to lockdown blues.

"Hi Doc, Can you call me asap?"

I called.

"I was losing a lot of hair, so I googled and found that it might be hypothyroidism. I checked thyroid, and you know what? It is abnormal".

Her thyroid-stimulating hormone (TSH) was above 10; I prescribed thyroxin supplement. Her fatigue disappeared as did her hair fall.

Both of us were happy—end of story.

I am happy because "*we*" arrived at the correct diagnosis.

The problem is that most often, neither the doctor nor the patient searches for an answer to a complex problem *together*.

This happens only when the doctor and the patient sit on the same side of the table, look at the same direction, and face the disease.

CHAPTER 15

Be Kind

Token number 37 turned out to be a 85-year-old lady with receding line of salt-pepper hair, socially distancing from the sand dune furrows of her forehead. Thinning, deforested eyebrows merging seamlessly with the countless radiating crow feet.

Seated in a wheelchair she smiled at me, a social smile quickly fading into oblivion by her obvious disability.

She must have had scores of admirers in her youth, I thought for a moment. Now her sole follower is a khaki-clad hospital orderly, pushing the wheelchair.

"Namastey", she wished me with folded hands and smiled.

The professional "white-coat" doctor in me returned the smile; the best I could produce at 3 in the afternoon.

"So, tell me how are you". I wanted to get back to business as fast as possible.

Makkal aharam kazhicho? Did you have lunch my son?

The person who used to ask me this same question with similar concern stopped asking sometime back. My mother lost her memory a decade before she died of Alzheimer's disease.

As the nurses helped her to my examination table, I could see the straps of her artificial legs—a double amputee.

You do not need to drive a Rolls Royce, you do not even need to walk on your own legs to make your doctor smile.

CHAPTER 16

Stab the Lab

"Doctor, I just went for a routine checkup and see what result your hospital lab has given me".

She dropped the sheaf of reports on my table like a dirty tissue paper.

It showed that her sugars were astronomically high.

"What a bad lab, they gave me a high sugar report".

It sounded as if the laboratory had a grudge against her and benefited by handing out a high blood sugar report.

I politely convinced her to repeat the tests.

Once the repeat reports confirmed the "sweet malady", she shifted the blame to her "previous" doctor.

"That doctor gave me some medicine for high blood pressure 3 years back, and that must be responsible for my diabetes. Of course, I didn't take those medicine for more than a month"!

The fact that none of her family members ever had diabetes confirmed that the poor doctor's "pressure medicine" is certainly the culprit. The doctor in question happened to be the best outgoing student in our senior batch in medical college.

My consultation room air conditioner suddenly felt so inadequate.

CHAPTER 17: Memory Test

"Doctor, do you remember me?" The patient asked.

I tried to log into the deepest vaults of my memory but this man's face looked unfamiliar.

So I try to impress him with my professional smile.

He does not budge.

"So tell me doc, you can't remember me? Just try".

I nod, a 5° bidirectional pendular nod, which could mean anything, from a solid yes or a volatile no depending on which side of Vindhyas you come from.

"So, could you tell me about your problem". I try to get back to business.

But Mr memory-checker will not budge.

"Well, well, doctor you can't remember me, right, shall I give you a clue. We met at the Airport".

"Ohh yes yes, and that was..."

"So I see, you can remember now? It was around 6 years back at the...".

I have a poor memory, and if that is what you are trying to test, I give up. At 2:30 pm, another 12 patients waiting to be consulted, my lunch box is still cooling its heels; it is not a good environment for an MCQ examination. But if you would rather tell me about your medical problem, I would try to solve it out.

Fortunately, voices in the head are too low in decibel scale to be heard.

Yes, Yes, anyway can we start with your medical problem?

Like a schoolteacher, a doctor meets hundreds of people. A doctor must get close to a person in order to obtain his personal, social, and family history to make a diagnosis and plan a treatment right for the patient. By trying to ask him questions regarding his memory just complicates things for the man in white coat.

If at all you want to start off with a familiarity platform, start off by telling, "we actually met at Mumbai airport, and introduced by Mr ABC our common friend".

I have some patients with high IQ who have already figured out my poor grades in the memory test. They start the conversation with a statement, "doctor we meant just about a month back and I am sure you can't remember". I actually don't remember and I don't mind.

The sole reason why the patient visits a doctor is to get a right diagnosis and a correct treatment. And the time is ticking away. There is no point in trying to put the doctor in an awkward position.

CHAPTER 18: Old Records

"So what medicines are you on?"

"The same that you wrote last time."

"And when was that?"

"I suppose 2019."

"Do you have the list?"

"No."

"Do you know the medicine names?"

"I can't remember."

I check the hospital record. He has taken a new registration.

"What happened to your old OP number?"

May be his dog chewed it, or whatever; but without knowing his medicine list, how do I alter it?

My handwriting is poor, illegible. But that scribble is important for your treatment. No expensive mounting, no rosewood frame, no lamination. Just keep a photo in your phone.

Recently, a patient told me that he is not sure about his medicines, but his wife has noted down the names of medicines. On our advice, he called home and wrote down the names and handed them over to us with a grin of showing of a hunting trophy.

My resident doctor took the paper and broke out in a laughter.

It read Cipla, Pfizer, and Merck, names of three leading pharma companies, each manufacturing hundreds of different brands of medicine. His wife wrote down the most prominently displayed word on the medicine strip.

— ♦ ♦ ♦ —

Medical records are extremely important for the doctor to make a diagnosis, chart your response to therapy, and move forward. Medication dosage are sometimes decreased or increased because of side effects or clinical response. Those are often noted in the prescription in a handwriting illegible to most but enough to give a vital clue to your doctor.

CHAPTER 18: Old Records

Once a patient came to the OPD with a thyroid function test report, which clearly showed features of hypothyroid, asking me to start medicines, since most of his family members were hypothyroid. "Now I too have become one", he commented. "Can I start with 25 or straight go to 50 micrograms?", he asked.

He was unhappy when we asked him to bring the list of medicines that he was taking, but the medicine list brought the next day showed that he was on a medicine called Amiodarone which alters thyroid function mimicking hypothyroid.

Another patient asked in a hushed voice if he can take Viagra once in a while. On detailed questioning it turned out that he was on nitrate pills (a pill for heart pain)—a strictly no-no combination, which could result in precipitous and often lethal drop of blood pressure.

Show a simple photo of the prescription in your cell phone to your grumpy doctor and his face would light up as if he was watching a funny TikTok video.

―◆◆◆―

"I have come for an opinion".

"I had a little chest pain, it is gone now. The local doctor took an ECG, suspected some heart disease. I want a full check-up, ECG, Echo Angio whatever".

"Could you show me the old ECG?"

"It is at home. I thought anyway we will have all these repeated".

The patient does not realize that a subtle ECG change during the pain, which has normalized now, could be my biggest clue to a diagnosis.

Please bring all your old reports when you go for a second opinion. It may be extremely important.

Please, for your sake.

CHAPTER 19

Bystanders

The patient was brought into the emergency room (ER) with cardiac arrest. He was promptly intubated and connected to a ventilator, but his vitals were bad. He had no urine output, low BP, and outcome looked bleak. He had a chest discomfort for 3 days; he ascribed it to gas and refused medical attention till the heart could take no more of it.

I called the bystanders.

He is very bad, unstable, pulse feeble, BP not recordable, and on a ventilator support. He is unable to breathe by himself. His kidneys too seem to be failing.

The young man listened carefully.

Finally, he looked up and said, "No other problem na doctor?"

I am unaware of any problem than a man's brain, heart, lungs, and kidney shutting down; I keep quiet.

I repeat the whole statement again slowly, hopeful that the seriousness would sink in this time. It seems it did. The young man looks at me; his eyes shine for a fraction of a second.

"Doctor, I am his neighbor, can I call his son so that you can directly explain him."

I still stand there, hanging on to the cliff.

The son comes in, I explain it again.

He understands the seriousness.

After a moment of silence, he says, "Doctor, could you please talk to my sister who is in the US who could understand it?"

He dials the number as I anxiously wait.

"Is your sister a doctor or a health worker?"

"No sir, but she has many doctor friends."

Patient management algorithms are very robust. They account for most variations encountered in clinical practice.

An entire session on bystander management is badly needed.

CHAPTER 20: Gossip

"You know doc; I know your dad so well, but it is years since we met. How's he?"

"He passed away 6 years back".

"Ohh really, I am so sorry, time flies you see".

"One Mr Satheesh used to always talk about your dad".

"So tell me what brings you here today", I try to course-correct.

"Well, I will tell you, but you know what? We are mentally strong, so small problems don't matter to us. This young generation—smoking, drinking….. I give up".

My OPD nurse slightly tilts her head pointing to the display board, stuck at token number 23.

Like every professional, your doctor is busy.

He too loves gossip and small talk over a cup of coffee but with a crowded OPD on a Monday with 28 more patients to be seen before the evening rounds, he is perhaps not in a proper frame of mind.

CHAPTER 21: Tests and More Tests

PRETEST PROBABILITY

Thomas Bayes belonged to Kent County in southern England and was known for his religious bent. He wrote two books in his lifetime. One named "Divine *benevolence*", a purely religious one, while the other was titled "An Introduction to the *Doctrine* of Fluxion". This second book was a treatise on mathematics of probability. It was only in 1763, 2 years after his death, when British philosopher Richard Price read the essays from this book at the Royal Society of London that the impact of the concept was really understood. The theory said that a "pretest probability" determines the post-test result. It is called Bayes theorem.

"Doctor, I am working in Dubai. I have no complaint as such but I want a full body scan", announced the overweight young man. The thick gold bracelet and the imported sunglass indicated that he is one of those successful nonresident Indians who have made a mark on the desert sand.

Today's medical world is dominated by technology. Tests ranging from CT scans, MRI scans, PET scans, angiograms, isotope studies, perfusion tests, to all high-tech cutting-edge technologies are easily available. These technologies let the physician see deep inside the human body, access the anatomy and physiology, and detect an abnormality much before it progresses to a major catastrophe. Most of these tests are safe and painless. Of course, they are costly, but apart from that, why not do it for everyone who can afford it? This question has been asked in Western societies where cost of medical therapy is not an individual headache but the onus of the insurance company. In a detailed analysis published in the British Medical Journal last year, different strategies of screening were tried in the society to see how effective they are. Surprisingly, high-tech screening, like scans and blood markers, did no better than a general screening strategy. This confirmed the notion that medical investigations have to be goal directed and not random screening.

A CT scan of head may turn out to be normal in Alzheimer's disease or migraine, where a simple clinical history may point to the correct diagnosis. Similarly, an angiogram may be normal in cardiomyopathy (a heart muscle disease) or pericarditis (an ailment of the protective cover of the heart). The point is, simply because it is high tech, it may not be able to pick out a disease.

However, a "pretest probability" changes it all. A 75-year- old man with history of diabetes, high blood pressure, and high cholesterol with a slight discomfort of the jaw and chest, on walking uphill, may indicate a block in the coronary artery (angina pectoris) and indicate an urgent need for an angiogram, while a 30-year-old lady with a severe chest pain in a localized point recurring only at bedtime is likely to be a noncardiac gastric ailment.

Biostatistics tells us that tests with low false negativity are the one, which are used as a screening tool while those with low false positive are reserved to clinch the diagnosis. If you do not follow the sequence, you are likely to go wrong all the way. That is what Thomas Bayes theorized and it holds good even today. The American College of Cardiology has now published the appropriateness criteria for tests to be applied in a particular complaint. A physician is free to decide who needs which test but in most cases, these guidelines need to be followed to prioritize investigations logically and save cost.

The next time your doctor spends more time asking you about your complaint or examine you in detail, rather than ordering a scan or a laboratory test, do not think he is wasting your time. Appreciate his knowledge and respect for the 250-year-old theory of a humble monk from England who taught us the correct way to arrive at an accurate diagnosis faster albeit at a lesser cost.

CHAPTER 22 | Diagnosis: Yours or Mine?

Many people come and consult me just to make me tell *what they believe they have.*

— ◆ ◆ ◆ —

"I have this chronic digestion problem and acidity for long, and I know this chest discomfort is nothing but gas. My wife insisted that I get it confirmed by you".

— ◆ ◆ ◆ —

"The other doctor really scared me saying that I might have some heart disease. He wrongly prescribed some medicines too; of course, I have stopped taking them after a month. Just wanted to get a checkup from you; I know you are the best".

— ◆ ◆ ◆ —

"The lab report showed that I have high blood sugar, which is impossible because I don't take sugar and no one in my family has diabetes. Also, I know that diabetes pills can damage the kidneys, and can increase blood pressure".

— ◆ ◆ ◆ —

"I have this chest discomfort on walking uphill. So, I got a heart scan done, and it is normal. Just wanted you to see these and confirm".

— ◆ ◆ ◆ —

Your wife, the other doctor, the laboratory reports, or the scan may be perfectly normal or grossly deranged, and you may be fighting fit or riddled with disease. Why not we work together in trying to make an *unbiased* diagnosis. Transferring your *bias* on to your doctor might give you a diagnosis that you want to hear but may not be correct one and good for you in the long run. Sometimes, a correct *early* diagnosis of a bad disease can have a better outcome compared to an undiagnosed low-grade disease, in the long run.

If you have come to show off your medical knowledge, you are welcome.

If you want my opinion, let us start from zero.

"Tell me how exactly you feel"
(Many patients do not like it at all when I do not look at their "expensive" reports *until* I take their detailed medical history and examine them clinically).

"So tell me about your problem".

"I have no problem at all but have come to see you at the insistence of my wife", he gently points to a saree-clad lady. I have this "gas" coming up to my chest as a walk and goes away as I stop. I know that it is a digestion problem, but she refuses to believe me. I am sure it is gas. Please convince her that I have no heart problem. Once you tell her, she would be convinced".

Go to your doctor with any symptoms and tell him all your complaints, your past history, everything. But do not force him to make a diagnosis that you think is right. Because, exactly like this gentleman who turned out to have multiple blockages of his coronary arteries, ending up finally in bypass surgery, forcing the doctor to make a diagnosis that you think is right may not always be good for you.

Our fear of a disease often makes us go in a diametrically opposite mode of denial and feel safe. We try to ascribe a cardiac pain to gas, a headache to a wrong diet, high blood pressure to a salty food, and diabetes to the ice-cream you had taken a week back.

While all these could cause alterations in symptoms and blood biochemistry, it is safe to rule it out.

CHAPTER 23
Criticizing the Previous Doctor

—◆◆◆—

"But sir, my previous doctor diagnosed me with heart ailment, isn't it wrong? And you find me absolutely healthy. I think that doctor is bad".

"I can tell you my opinion about your disease but cannot comment about his", is my stock answer.

—◆◆◆—

Appreciation of his work and crediting him for a right diagnosis certainly makes a doctor happy. In the same breath, many patients feel that criticizing other doctors and belittling them make the current doctor happy.

—◆◆◆—

"A patient who criticizes the previous doctor will do the same about you to the next doctor", my professor had told me once, and I believe that it is very true.

—◆◆◆—

Lyn–Flynn effect indicates that in every generation, average IQ increases, needing to upgrade the metrics of IQ measurements. This means, your next-generation doctors are going to be smarter and better. Accept that earlier, the better. So, a younger doctor might pick out a disease that you did not suspect. The doctor reflexively assumes it to be a bad thing that he had failed to suspect a disease. In contrast, as long as you are a team with the patient, it is good news for the patient. So when my old patient whom we were treating for a long time with progressive breathlessness and no clue to the reason for worsening, referred to the chest physician for a fiberoptic bronchoscopy, came running to my OPD, fought with my OPD nurse, squeezed inside past waiting patients, to break the good news that he has tuberculosis with a cure in sight, that is because to him we are a team, and as joyous as his family. Not sulking a bit, because we have failed to pick it up.

We won, as a team.

CHAPTER 24
Minor Irritants, Loss of Focus

"Your token display systems are bad".
"I think you need to have more chairs".
"The pharmacy is too crowded".

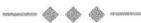

Traditionally, the doctor is the face of medicine, and it includes everything, from services to diagnosis to cleanliness and administration. But now times have changed. The doctor in a large multispecialty hospital is a part of a whole system. He is an employee, a cog in the process.

It is not wrong for you to complain about such trivia to the doctor; in fact, it is very likely that he will forward it to the admin and the admin would take action, far more swiftly than your review in Google. During your next visit, you are likely to see a better display or more seating space. But the single most important reason for your visiting the doctor is not to get the seating space right but a right diagnosis and the right direction. Loading him with trivial complaints do not help you and might take his focus off. Let the doctor apply his mind to your diagnosis and not spend his time and energy on conveniences and services.

On your way out, ask for the PRO and put in all your complaints and suggestions. The seats may still remain cramped, but you might get a better diagnosis and direction.

Focus

"After you see me, I would request you to see my wife also. She did not get an appointment today".

Your focus is to get a proper diagnosis for you, and that is why you are waiting to consult the doctor. He must focus, concentrate, and make a right assessment, order tests, and interpret them. Finally, he has to provide you with a direction. Do not take away his focus by introducing problems that distract him.

CHAPTER 25

Emotional Blackmail, Warranty

"Okay doctor, so I understand that angioplasty and stenting will cure the block. And that should guarantee that there would be no problem at all in the future".

—◆◆◆—

"I hope the medicines that you write will have no side effects. I have heard that blood-pressure medicines damage the kidneys".

—◆◆◆—

"Doctor, I don't want to listen to all those medical terms, I don't understand them. I give you a free hand. All I want is to get back my mother, walking around, healthy as before".

—◆◆◆—

"But doctor she came walking to the hospital".

—◆◆◆—

Doctors practice medicine, but medical practice has its limitations. No amount of money, fame, power, or contact can undo a bad health condition. Despite having sufficient wealth and access to best health care, Steve Jobs died prematurely of pancreatic cancer. World leaders, top businessmen, film personalities die of stroke, heart disease, cancer or get debilitated by Alzheimer's disease, for no fault of theirs.

The doctor can, at best, treat the disease with the best available evidence-based medicine but cannot ensure a good outcome or guarantee a cure in every case.

There is no guarantee of good health after a complex procedure, no drug that is free of side effects. Simply because a patient looks well, dressed in costly attire, or comes in walking does not mean that he is healthy inside.

CHAPTER 26
Medical Jargon and Acronym

Probably it was the need for safety and confidentiality that most high-level petitions, applications, and communications were written in a language understood only by the select few; priests addressed the Gods in *Hebrew, Urdu,* or *Sanskrit*; software specialists wrote computer applications in *Java*; while doctors communicated in Greek and Latin. This restricted the understanding of such subjects only to eligible candidates. It also brought about a halo of exclusivity and an aura of mystery to those standing inside the elite circle, transacting in what sounded like jargon to others.

Doctors used medical jargons for justifiable reasons. During rounds, at the bedside he could not pronounce that the patient would shortly die; in contrast, a statement like *"guarded prognosis"* sounded so cultured. *"Idiopathic"* implied that the doctor was at a loss as to what the diagnosis could be, while *"therapeutic trial"* meant that he is shooting in the dark. Finally, when the doctor exhausted all his options, and the patient all his money, he was offered *"symptomatic palliative"* treatment.

Everyone knows that doctors love alphabets, the more the merrier. Like school children playing the word game "scrabble", they compete with each other trying to get a longer degree, everything from A to Z, leaving little space in their name board, and little doubt in the patient's mind regarding the doctor's academic excellence. The long list of alphabets may not be useful in curing the patient's pain, but helps to impress the bystanders, so that even if the disease refuses to go, the weight of those alphabets would shift the weight in favor of the doctor.

Over time, doctors started converting common words to acronyms, not just to impress a patient, but even to derogate a technology. When "stent implantation" emerged as a new technology, proving it to be better than the traditional "balloon angioplasty", doctors quickly named it as "plain old balloon angioplasty" (POBA). POBA is a standard acronym today, even in medical textbooks.

— ♦ ♦ ♦ —

The other day, I was listening to a young doctor trying to educate an elderly couple about the prospects of a heart bypass surgery.

SECTION 2: Real Life

"I think *CABG* (coronary artery bypass surgery) is a better option than *PCI* (percutaneous coronary angioplasty) especially that there are some *tandem lesions*, one *bifurcation lesion* and one *CTO* (chronic total occlusion), do you understand what I mean?"

The wide-eyed, white-haired lady responded with a typical South-Indian nod, which could mean anything; her husband did not, perhaps his spondylitis-laden stiff neck prevented him from doing so.

Their son, listening intently, remained silent for 10 seconds and then asked, "so doctor, there is no other major problem?"

Medical terms and acronyms, transacted from doctor to patient, created confusion but now the roles have reversed; the doctor is getting it back with compound interest.

— ♦ ♦ ♦ —

Larry Page and Sergey Brin never imagined that their creation "Google" would bring jargons and acronyms out of the four walls of the hospital, to the common man's bedroom. Here are some examples as to how it leads to misuse of medical jargons.

— ♦ ♦ ♦ —

"Doctor, my reports say that I have enlarged ventricles", the patient paused.

The ventricle of the heart is the main pumping chamber, and enlargement of this important element of heart is a major problem, needing rest and restriction of activities.

Before I could find words to convey the grave outcome, the patient threw the bombshell.

"My doctor told me to do exercise and more sudoku".

I was stunned for a moment, but quickly remembered that the brain also had a ventricle and that too could enlarge leading to dementias.

— ♦ ♦ ♦ —

"Doctor, *cabbage* didn't work for me, so they opted for *plus-tea*".

As a cardiologist, I realize that he is talking about CABG and angioplasty and not about nutritional advice, but an ophthalmologist may not be aware about it.

MR means mitral regurgitation (a valve leak) to the cardiologist, mental retardation to the neurologist, and medial rectus (an eye muscle) to an ophthalmic surgeon.

— ♦ ♦ ♦ —

CHAPTER 26: Medical Jargon and Acronym

Superspecialization makes a doctor expert in a niche area, but, as a result, more myopic; often, our knowledge of *acronym* is much less than the google-searching patient who is reading everything about just one problem; his own. While as a cardiologist I play with terms like CABG and angioplasty, the neurologist and the ophthalmologist have their own ABCD, and I am not always sure what they mean.

The stylish package of medical "jargon" that doctors were using so long to amaze and astound the poor patient has been now thrown back at the doctor, with devastating effects.

It is like switching on to bright light, if your opposing motorist does not dim. It does not teach him a lesson but increases the chance of a head-on collision.

A confused patient can relearn. A confused doctor can also relearn, but it may be too late. Let the medical jargon go back to where it came from—the doctor's brown bag.

Till then, let us talk about your problems in a language that both of us are proficient and comfortable.

CHAPTER 27

Medicine Dosage

■ CASE 1

Folded hands, dhoti and shirt, age 70 years

Language Malayalam

"Sir, please write a mild dose, my wife doesn't tolerate strong allopathic medicines. Normally I give her homeo".

■ CASE 2

GAP shirt, Levi's faded blue denim, i-Phone Pro falling out of pocket

Language English

"Hi doc you changed the diabetic medication of 1 mg of glimepiride to 1000 mg of metformin. I was just wondering if it was a mistake of sorts, or do you think I need a dose escalation of like 1000 times?"

■ CASE 3

Saree, school teacher

Language Malayalam

"I take insulin only in the morning and my random blood sugar level is normal. My HbA1c is 11%, but I think that's because I had taken some ladoo last week. I don't tolerate twice daily insulin".

Vastly different cultural background, education, and knowledge but same thought process. Strong medicine, high dose.

Logically, higher dose is stronger, works more, and has more side effects. But somehow this logic *does not hold good always* in medicine.

The common insulin (Mixtard 30/70) has an effect duration of 8–10 hours and needs to be taken twice a day mostly, unless supplemented by other tablets or insulin. A glycated hemoglobin (HbA1c) of >6.5% is a signal of poor sugar control. *Suboptimal dose is ineffective.* 1 mg of glimepiride may produce more lowering of sugar level (stronger) than 1,000 mg of metformin. Every medicine has a biological half-life which determines how long it will be effective when a single dose is administered. Taking a tablet with a half-life of 6 hours every alternate day will have no beneficial effect. Similarly, each drug has an optimal therapeutic blood level which is determined by the amount of medicine absorbed, metabolism by the liver, and excretion by the kidneys. So, 1 g of a particular chemical may not necessarily be 1,000 times more effective than another medication at 1 mg dose.

Aspirin was first isolated from tree bark as a painkiller. Purified, and acetylated, salicylic acid hit the market, and quickly got into every American closet. An accidental finding by a surgeon that his patients on aspirin were bleeding more made him undertake trials that found out that aspirin had an anticlotting effect as well. But there was something unusual. Low dose of aspirin between 50 and 150 mg daily had this "blood thinning" effect, while it disappeared when high dose was administered. High-dose aspirin inhibited an additional enzyme in the vascular endothelium that neutralized its anticlotting effect. The aspirin that you take for *prevention of heart disease is a much lower dose* than that used to counter chronic arthritis.

Many drugs are effective for a particular disease only when used in low dose. *Rivaroxaban*, an anticlotting medicine (dose 15 mg), is used in irregular heart rhythm [atrial fibrillation (AF)] to prevent stroke. Studies have shown that when it is used in low dosage (2.5 mg twice daily) it prevents heart attacks and lower-limb vascular episodes. *Low-dose statins* for prevention of heart disease in diabetes, low-dose Aldactone and digoxin for heart failure, *low-dose methotrexate* (an anticancer drug) for arthritis, the list goes on and on.

Albert Hofmann working in Swiss Lab synthesized a new chemical, a di-ethyl-amide of lysergic acid (LSD). He took a small (huge by today's standard) dose of 250 µg and cycled home. It was then that he experienced the "acid trip" for the first time. A feel that his mind left his body with colorful hallucinations was something never described before. Over time, LSD became the psychedelic agent of choice for those who wanted to experience such "trips". Despite reports that some have never come back to normal after such "drug trips", LSD is still considered not addictive, and safe. The experience of bright light, bizarre shapes, nonexistent images, and the *mind*

leaving the body has lured many youngsters to try it, at a dose much lower (100 µg). Supporters of LSD point to the fact that despite several years of use, Hofmann himself lived up to the age of 102 years as a testimony to the safety of LSD.

But today a very *low dose* of 10 µg is now being tried for several diseases like terminal cancer pain, anxiety neurosis, and post-traumatic stress disorder (PTSD).

—◆◆◆—

There are different doses that work for different people, different body weight, and gender. Some need low dose, some need high dose.

A doctor does not gain anything by writing 5 or 50 mg of a dose nor does he get any thrill out of giving multiple injections. He is happy if your illness abates.

While *you* view illness as a pain, discomfort, fever, or cough (*symptoms*), the *doctor* is bothered about *disease progression*. An uncontrolled sugar, a persistent high pressure, or clotting tendency may create problem in the long run. The "high" "strong" dose is directed at preventing such unseen future problems. In contrast, situations that need low dose *need only low dose* and do not respond to high dose.

CHAPTER 28

Walking-in

People try their best to somehow avoid meeting a "white coat" but we get stressed out at the sight of a bunch of colors—"black coat", "khaki uniform", and "white and white" waiting in our outpatient department (OPD). While lawyers and police are easy to handle, politicians in "white and white" are a different level altogether.

—◆◆◆—

This 50-year-old "district level leader" apparently came for a routine checkup. Claiming to be a borderline diabetic, his blood sugar showed 445 mg% and his BP levels were so high that it made ours shoot up.

After the "ECG? Why ECG?" argument, the ECG was taken. That is when our adrenaline surged.

ECG showed severe diffuse STT changes suggestive of ischemia. Troponin was positive indicating ongoing cardiac damage. We advised an immediate coronary angiogram, which his family agreed after a lot of haggling.

A critical lesion in the proximal left anterior descending (LAD) artery was detected and immediate angioplasty advised, as a lifesaving measure. On the cath-table, before the procedure, he had a ventricular tachycardia (VT; cardiac arrest). He was defibrillated. A quick angioplasty was done; he was revived but remained on a ventilator in the intensive coronary care unit (ICCU).

Then the questioning started.

Barrage of phone calls. Not just anxiety, sympathy, shock, or sigh of relief, but doubt about the need for the procedure.

One young "white and white" gentleman walks in.

"But doctor, he came walking", was the main argument.

"Yes, he did".

"And after your treatment now he is on a ventilator".

"Yes".

"He had a major block in the main artery. We had to try to clear it on an emergency basis…."

He was distracted as his mobile phone rang, he picked it up.

"Minister calling….." he said in a hushed tone, winked and walked away. He never came back.

The progression of a disease is called its "natural history". Many diseases remain silent for a while before they show their colors. A tumor in the abdomen, elevated blood sugar, or cholesterol may not cause any discomfort (aka *symptoms*). A diabetic may present with a silent heart attack but feel nothing—again no *symptom (asymptomatic)*. When a patient has minimal or no symptoms, he comes to medical attention often for a routine checkup or some vague mild complaints.

Sometimes, such patients may feel nothing but may harbor a life-threatening disease, but the patient may not be aware of it.

Medical treatments are mostly safe but can have side effects, mostly minor. But procedures, like a surgery or an angioplasty, have their own risk. But the procedure is undertaken because the *benefits outweigh the risk by a huge margin*. More importantly, a natural history event—"a cardiac arrest" or a "stroke"—can come *any time during a treatment*. At *home or hospital*, whether he comes in walking, crawling, driving, or unconscious in a trolley does not make a difference.

The doctor is not necessarily responsible for the *natural history of a disease* or for the *standard side effects of a procedure*. Scare of adverse consequences would deter the doctor from delivering the right treatment, especially in an *asymptomatic, critical illness, needing a high-risk intervention*.

I fear the statement, "But he came walking".

I fear asymptomatic patients walking into my OPD with a critical disease, needing an intervention.

CHAPTER 29
Allergy

"Doctor, please write a medicine that doesn't produce allergy".
Unfortunately, there is none.

—◆◆◆—

During a cruise in 1901, Prince Albert of Monaco suggested to the two scientists, Charles Richet and Paul Portier, to look into effects of jellyfish toxin. They tried to immunize dogs with small-dose injection of the toxin and produce resistance. To their surprise, they found that dogs exposed previously to a small dose of toxin reacted badly to the second dose and died. They called this phenomenon as anaphylaxis (ana—again; phylaxis—protection).

Anaphylaxis is the worst kind of allergy that can instantly kill unless emergency treatment is rendered.

Allergic reactions can range from mild itching or running nose after exposure to pollen grains to sudden collapse after a penicillin injection. The source may vary, from peanuts to penicillin, from skin cream to seafood. It is always safe to note the name of the drug that you are allergic to. Unlike what people believe, there is no allergy-free drug. Individuals react to drugs, not the other way round. It is always wise to carry a record of drugs that you are allergic to, so that the doctor makes sure that his prescription does not include a similar chemical.

—◆◆◆—

"Doctor let me tell you one thing, I am allergic to all medicines, that's why I take only natural medicines".

I am still not sure why I am seeing this patient.

—◆◆◆—

CHAPTER 30

Fake News

First few days at school, your little angel cries incessantly, refusing to go, despite the glamor of uniform and school bag; by the end of the week, she starts making friends and by week 2, she learns the first bad "swear" word. She spells it out loudly, not to embarrass you, but confirming her innocence and lack of knowledge about the intended audience who would enjoy it.

Sharing unusual, abnormal, attractive stuff is human instinct. And that is where the problem starts.

As a doctor, I had never come across a mom who says that her kid eats well, a wife who says that her husband listens to her advice, and a nonresident software professional who thinks that his parents are not stubborn.

I have no answer as to why a kid should not enjoy drinking tasteless milk or bland vegetables, or a husband asking for an extra cup of coffee despite detected to have a borderline blood pressure, or why a 70-year-old lady would refuse to go and settle down in the land of "gun-and-honey", especially when a wheelchair transfer is arranged, but I had to stammer and answer these questions all along my career.

But there is change in the air. In the last one decade of my cardiology practice, I find change in the pattern of questions that patients ask, not because of a happier mom, a contended wife, or a satisfied son, but because of a bright luminous LCD screen taking over all our lives, the cellphone—the ultimate device to find and share unusual, attractive but senseless stuff.

The game in the phone makes the kid eat even the blandest diet, while the mom is scrolling the Facebook looking for likes and the father texting his friends. The NRI son can make a videocall any time and see that the imported walking stick is in use. But that is not the issue here.

The doctor now has a new problem and that needs to be underscored—it is fake news.

Dr John W Krooner, MD, Mayo Clinic, has said that cholesterol is no longer a problem. Dr Baxter K Rosenbaum published his research that blood pressure pills are responsible for many deaths in Canada. A miniature device, the size of a matchbox, can now purify blood, thus avoiding the need for dialysis, and is soon going to be available in New Zealand. Researchers at the Institute of

Health Science at Baltimore found that use of flour *(maida)* in Indian food is the real reason for majority of cancer in India.

All these news came to my social media feed (WhatsApp) today, forwarded by my patients, asking me for my opinion. I am in the editorial board of half-a-dozen international medical journals but have never come across such news. To most Indians, a western name, attached to a high-sounding institute, impresses them so much that they fail to confirm their veracity. All of these are fake medical news; the doctor names, their institute credentials, the information—all fake.

Even if they are untrue, sharing them is fun, right? Wrong.

Reports that a new technique can easily avoid bypass, or taking medicines for an illness like hypertension or diabetes might damage kidneys, is more damaging to an individual than a political rhetoric. For the sharer, it is fun, but for the person waiting for a bypass surgery tomorrow, such a news may confuse him to take a wrong and costly decision.

Why not put a statutory warning *"social media medical information may be injurious to health"*? I asked one of my friends who is a software professional.

"Yes, good idea; we call it 'clickbait'". He smiled. "Actually such notifications, on the contrary, attract more visitors and more hits", he added.

These fake news are of no value. Do not forward them to your doctor, in a bid to educate him. Everyday I get scores of them forwarded to me as "...doctor are you aware about this new development?" Doctors get information about new development through respected medical journals, not social media/WhatsApp.

Do not waste your important 5 minutes starting with "...so doctor, you must have read that in US now cholesterol is no longer considered bad".

Section 3

To-do List

CHAPTER 31

Dress

In most western hospitals, the patient needs to change dress to a green hospital tunic, for the doctor to examine with ease and comfort, without disturbing your modesty and privacy. The outpatient department (OPD) of Indian hospitals lets the patient wear their own dress and partly undress as necessary. Privacy settings are at the minimal level in many government setups, so plan well before your appointment. Wear a loose-fitting dress that is easy to take off in case you need to change to hospital tunic. A two-piece dress is ideal since it is easy to undress. Remember that the changing rooms in hospitals are not spacious. Wear a clean set of undergarments; it is embarrassing being caught with a dirty bullet-hole ridden vest. It is better to avoid heavy makeup and nail polish because it makes detection of anemia or cyanosis (blue discoloration because of low oxygen levels) difficult. Too much of jewelry and tight-fitting dress are better avoided for the purpose of inconvenience and safe keeping. For women, an accompanying lady bystander would be nice if you are planning for a gynecology checkup. Remember that privacy is a right in the hospital, as is an explanation prior to any investigation or procedure. No good doctor is perturbed or angry at your asking for an explanation of what test you are supposed to undergo. Also understand that hospital staff are under immense stress in view of their nature of work. It is not unusual for some of them to act cold to your query.

FOOD, DRINK, COFFEE

Take a light breakfast or a brunch before you go, because hospital appointments are notorious for delays and might spring up some surprises and eventually unforeseen investigations like a scan. A short surgical procedure may need you to have a light diet. Carry a bottle of drinking water, especially if you are planning for an ultrasound scan of the abdomen.

Most hospital waiting areas have coffee kiosks; I strongly recommend against it. It is better to avoid caffeinated drinks since it might push up your blood pressure (BP) and heart rate, which are already prone to acceleration in view of hospital anxiety (white-coat hypertension). If you are a diabetic, carry some snacks (biscuits) or condiments in case you feel hypoglycemic.

SECTION 3: To-do List

■ STOPPING THE PILL

Do not stop your BP or diabetic medicine on the day of hospital visit, since the doctor wants to check how your numbers are while you are on the drugs. Many people stop the medicine on the pretext, "I will restart after seeing the doctor". This confuses the doctor since he is not sure as to why your BP is still high—is it because you skipped the medicines or is it that this drug is not working for you and need to be changed or dosage hiked?

■ MASK

When a doctor examines you, his physical proximity needs to be respected. As much as you do not want someone to cough or sneeze on your face, the same holds true for your doctor. In pediatric practice, most Indian mothers would fondly ask their kids to cough and "show" the doctor, and the kid coughs right at the doctor's face. The bacteria and virus unfortunately do not care about the qualification or the status or age of the next host.

Also, hospital is a place where people come with many illnesses, diagnosed and undiagnosed. Hospital-acquired "nosocomial" infections are much worse than those found in the community.

Have you heard of a Crab? Not the usual one. To the microbiologist, CRAB stands for Carbapenem-resistant *Acinetobacter baumannii*—a bacterium that is resistant to most antibiotics, known to man. Where do you find it? Well in the hospital. Despite the antiseptic stench, the handwash, the mask, the sanitizers in every nook and corner, hidden along those shiny doorknob and gleaming handrails, lurk deadly bacteria. The bacteria that you catch in a shopping mall would die of one of hundreds of antibiotics that we have with us, but hospital-acquired infections are a different ball game. It is true that only few of those who have a depressed immune system (not just HIV), like long-standing diabetes, or those on chemotherapy, including a viral infection, might temporarily suppress our immunity, making us more susceptible to bacterial infections.

A mask might be uncomfortable in the short term but wearing it to the hospital is always advisable.

■ MOBILE PHONE

As I start concentrating on the heart sounds, a Bollywood number or haunting music reminds me of a disco dance or a romantic scene. It is not very conducive for applying my mind on a cardiac diagnosis. Muting your cellphone saves a lot of irritation for both the doctor and the patient. I was once called to the court to give expert witness on a case. The lawyer told me that the Judge is very strict; if she hears a cellphone ring in the courtroom, she will direct the cellphone owner to reamin in the room as a punishment till the court is adjourned by evening. The doctor in his clinic cannot do that but an angry and upset doctor alters the whole game plan of a better diagnosis, the focus point of the exercise.

Hospital is no normal visiting place. Avoid taking very young children and very elderly people, unless they need a medical consultation themselves.

CHAPTER 32 | How to Select a Specialist?

How do we select a product in Amazon? We find the group and look at the options. The first thing we check is the star ratings; anything less than 4/5 is out. Then we check the reviews and finally the picture and click buy.

But this is not a good strategy in choosing your specialist.

The more famous, busy specialist may not be the best for you. We have an excellent neurosurgeon, very famous, magical hands. Since he is so famous, all patients with neurological problem (nonsurgical) flock to him, from Alzheimer's disease to vascular headache. And he is hesitant to say no to the patient, unable to tell him that he is not the best person to treat them. The result is poor prescription ending up in amusement of younger colleagues, but patients are proud to claim that they are under his treatment.

The best way out is ask an insider opinion, a family physician, a GP, or even a medical representative. In fact in India, medical representatives are a very reliable source of information because they cover many doctors, talk to their colleagues, and know who exactly is good in business.

Is the most famous doctor best for me?

I had a patient who wanted his angioplasty to be done by the best interventional cardiologist in the country, and we referred him to a top-notch interventional cardiologist. A week later, he came back and told me that he had got his procedure done by another *less-well-known* cardiologist of the same hospital. On asking the reason for change of mind, he said, "as the doctor was watching my angio, he was interrupted by phone calls from ministers and film stars, and he was unable to concentrate on my case. I went to this other 'less-known' doctor who took time, studied my case well, and explained everything. I let him do the procedure. Now I am fine".

Choose your specialist not just by name, fame, or length of his degrees. Look deeper. Spend enough time researching. Your life depends on his decision.

CHAPTER 33

Second Opinion

"Doctor, last week I went for the morning walk, and I met Dr ABC, he knows me, and asked me about my well-being. I told him that I am under your care, and he casually saw your prescription. He fully agreed with all you said and asked me to enquire if the dosage of... could be reduced?"

What surprises me is that how many of my patients bump into a senior cardiologist by accident in shopping malls and parks and get casually enquired about their medical prescription.

Asking for a second opinion is good; after all it is your health and well-being, and it is the single most important thing to you. But you do not need to tell me a story to do that.

Most modern doctors do not mind your taking a second opinion. If your doctor is on your side, both of you are fighting the same problem, he would tell you whether or not you need a second opinion. Please do not lie; the doctor might maintain a straight face, but he knows.

CHAPTER 34

Tools to Carry

"Any old reports?"
"No."
"Any old hospital record, old registration number, or a prescription?"
"No."

─── ♦♦♦ ───

Please carry all your medical records, prescriptions, laboratory reports, X-ray, ECG, scans everything, when you go to the hospital.

In 1927, Bluma Zeigarnik, a psychiatric resident in Berlin, went to a local restaurant for dinner with her friends. She was wearing a flaming red scarf around her neck, which really stood out. The waiter came to take the orders. As each one of the dozen students ordered, the waiter confirmed each order with a nod and finally went back to the kitchen. Zeigarnik noted that the waiter never jotted down the orders on a paper. When the food and drinks came in, the waiter served each one of them correctly with no mistakes. Zeigarnik was wonderstruck by the supermemory of the waiter. The group thanked him and left. A little later, Zeigarnik realized that she had left behind her scarf on the restaurant table and went back to collect it. She found the "supermemory" waiter and enquired about her scarf. To her surprise, the waiter failed to recognize her, let alone her scarf. When she enquired about his supermemory and the sequence of orders, he casually answered, "Oh, the orders? I just forget them after I serve." Zeigarnik effect indicates that once a task is done, the short-term human memory forgets it conveniently.

The doctor, exactly like the waiter, might have discussed everything about your illness, but it is unlikely that he would remember it after a week. He might vaguely remember, but such vagueness is not acceptable in medical practice.

The doctor or the heathcare staff cannot remember what your medical background is. They may be finally able to fish out your data, but the wastage of time and resource would divert the doctor's attention for a better diagnosis.

> "Let the doctor and the patient hold hands and travel together in search of the right diagnosis and direction of good health."

Index

A

Accidents 14
Aging gracefully in different ways 17
Algoritmi de numero Indorum 11
Allergic reactions 59
Alzheimer's disease 44
American College of Cardiology 45
Ammumma 14, 15
Anaphylaxis 59
Android app 12
Angiogram 5, 6, 18
Angioplasty 68
Anticancer drug 55
Anxiety neurosis 56
Arthritis 55
Aspirin 55
Attractive stuff 60
Awkward position 39

B

Back-lit scan report 5
Bacterium 66
Balloon angioplasty 51
  plain old 51
Berlin, psychiatric resident in 70
Blood biochemistry 47
Blood pressure 46, 65
Bored 15
Brain scan 23
Brownian movement 21
Bypass surgery 18
Bystander management 42

C

Carbapenem-resistant *Acinetobacter baumannii* 66
Cardiac arrest 57
Cardiac issue, complex 26
Cardiological Society of India 34
Cardiomyopathy 44
Cath-table 57
Cell phone 41
Cellular level 3
Chaos-prone health system 22
Chest
  discomfort 46
  pain 6, 41
Chilly morning 14
Chorea, case of 22
Complex signaling system 3
Constipation, chronic 10
Consultation room 37
Cough 56
Crash landings 14
Critical disease 58
Criticizing 48
Crossroads, options of 33
Cultural background 54
Culturally divergent group 19

D

Death sentences 5
Deforested eyebrows merging 36
Diabetic medication 54, 66
Diagnosis
  correct early 46
  right 39
  unbiased 46
Digestion problem, chronic 46
Direction 24, 26
  right 26
  thinking 26
Discomfort 10, 56
Disease
  cure 10
  fear of 47
  progression of 58
District level leader 57
Doc scare 33

Index

Doctors
   attention for better diagnosis 70
   deal with torn arms 8
   modern 69
   smile 36
Dress 65
   tight-fitting 65
Drug trips 55

E

Emergency room 29
Emotional blackmail, warranty 50
Epidemiology 10
Experimental therapy 9
Eye muscle 52

F

Fake news 60
Family physician 68
   specialization and loss of 12
Family reunion 14
Feel free 26
Feel hypoglycemic 65
Fever 6, 56
Fluxion, doctrine of 44
Focus 49
Food 65

G

Gas 31, 47
   diverse manifestations of 32
   laughing 32
   potato-induced 32
Glimepiride 54
Glycated hemoglobin 54
Gods in Hebrew 51
Good health, guarantee of 50
Gossip 43
Guarded prognosis 51

H

Hacking cough 10
Handwriting illegible 40
Headache 6, 23
   severe 10

Health worker 42
Heart disease in diabetes, prevention of 55
Heart
   protective cover of 45
   rate 65
   transplant 17
Heavy makeup 65
Heuristics 11
Hip replacement 4
Hospital record, old 70
Human body 8
Hypertension Council 34

I

Idiopathic 51
Illness 8, 16
Immune system 66
Immunize dogs 59
Indian attire, traditional 18
Indian health system 16
Indian hospitals lets 65
Injurious to health 61
Inside doctor's mind 10
Insulin 54
Intensive coronary care unit 15, 57
IQ measurements, metrics of 48
Irritating complaint 29

K

Kalahari heat 3
Kerb-side consult, right or wrong 20

L

Laboratory reports 46, 70
Lancet 20
Laughter 40
Legal binding 26
Lesion, bifurcation 52
Life
   quality 3
   real 27
Life-changing events 7
Lifesaving measure 57
Lyn–Flynn effect indicates 48
Lysergic acid, di-ethyl-amide of 55

M

Malayalam language 54
Mask 66
Maverick west 22
Medical
  acronym 51
  checkup 7
  consultation 67
  jargon 51, 53
  practice 50
  problem 38
  records 70
  school toughens 8
  therapy, aggressiveness of 19
  wonders, modern 3
Medicine
  dosage 54
  pressure 37
  teaches doctors, modern 9
Memory test 38
Metformin 54
Methyl isocyanate 31
Migraine 44
Mind, proper frame of 43
Minor irritants, loss of focus 49
Mitral regurgitation 52
Mobile phone 66
Movement disorder 22

N

Neurological problem 68
Numb toe 10

O

Ophthalmic surgeon 52
Opinion 24, 26
  second 69
Outpatient department 33, 65

P

Palliative, symptomatic 51
Pancytopenia 5
Papillary carcinoma 22
Percutaneous coronary angioplasty 52
Pericarditis 45
Philosophy 19
Pill, stopping 66
Placebo 29
Post-traumatic stress disorder 56
Prescription 70
Pretest probability 44
Professional smile 38
Proximal left anterior descending 57

R

Registration number, old 70
Religious rituals 17
Reuniting broken parts 10
Rivaroxaban 55
Romantic scene 66

S

Science 3
Setting stage 5
Sharing unusual 60
Siberian cold 3
Silicon Valley 17
Skin cream to seafood 59
Sniffer-dog-baiting 12
Soap-water 12
Social media
  feed 61
  medical information 61
Specialist, select 68
Stab lab 37
Stent implantation 51
Stomach pain 6
Stop kerb-side consultation 20
Stroke 58
Suboptimal dose 55
Supermemory 70
Surgery proceeded 15
Sweet malady 37
Swollen glands 23
Symptom relief 10

T

Tandem lesions 52
Teaching the doctor 34
Tests and more tests 44
Therapeutic trial 51
Thyroid
  cancer, type of 22
  function mimicking hypothyroid 41
  stimulating hormone 34

Index

Tiredness 6
Tools to carry 70
Traffic, two way 1
Tsunami, third 13

U

Ulcerative colitis 5
Undeniably robust 18

V

Valve leak 52
Ventricular tachycardia 57

W

Walking-in 57
WhatsApp 61
Wheelchair 36
White-coat hypertension 65

Z

Zeigarnik 70
  effect 70
  noted 70
  realized 70

EU GSPR Authorised Reprsentative
Logos Europe, 9 rue Nicolas Poussin
1700, La Rochelle, France
Phone: +33 (0) 6 67 93 73 78
E-mail: contact@logoseurope.eu

www.ingramcontent.com/pod-product-compliance
Ingram Content Group UK Ltd.
Pitfield, Milton Keynes, MK11 3LW, UK
UKHW060949220426
5322IPUK00033B/602